ADVANCE PRAISE FOR *HOW TO THINK LIKE A NEUROLOGIST*

"Meltzer's *How to Think Like a Neurologist* is even more than that—it's a masterful clinical handbook for learning how to tackle unknowns. What do you do if the diagnosis is not already obvious and there is no algorithm to follow? How do you tailor your history by asking probing questions that will help to refine hypotheses? And how do you refute your hypotheses through directed, customized neurological examinations? The syndromic approach beautifully elaborated by Meltzer is a prerequisite for delivering the kind of value-based and patient-centered care we all seek—and to do so one patient at a time."

—William J. Schwartz, MD, Assistant Dean for Faculty Affairs, Distinguished Teaching Professor, Professor and Associate Chair of Research & Education, Dept. of Neurology, Dell Medical School, The University of Texas at Austin

"*How to Think Like a Neurologist* presents a clear, practical approach to clinical reasoning in neurology. Working step by step through a series of real-world cases, Dr. Meltzer uses a conversational style to elucidate the principles of neurologic diagnosis. This is essential reading for students on their neurology rotation, residents in neurology, and any medical provider seeking to improve their understanding of clinical neurology."

—Aaron Berkowitz, MD, PhD, Professor of Neurology, Kaiser Permanente, Los Angeles, CA and author of *Clinical Neurology and Neuroanatomy: A Localization-Based Approach*

"Finally, a book that captures the intangibles of neurologic diagnosis. The synthetic ability that combines knowledge of how diseases affect the nervous system, personal clinical experience, and systematic inquiry is on display. Nowhere do these qualities come together more obviously than in neurology. By analyzing clinical cases that delve into the inner workings of a master clinician, Meltzer has provided a terrific contribution to pedagogy and to clinical work in the field."

—Alan Ropper, MD, Department of Neurology, Brigham and Women's Hospital, Boston, MA

HOW TO THINK LIKE
A NEUROLOGIST

A Case-Based Guide to
Clinical Reasoning in Neurology

Ethan Meltzer, MD

ASSISTANT PROFESSOR
DEPARTMENT OF NEUROLOGY
THE UNIVERSITY OF TEXAS AT AUSTIN DELL MEDICAL SCHOOL

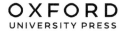

OXFORD
UNIVERSITY PRESS

Oxford University Press is a department of the University of Oxford. It furthers the University's objective of excellence in research, scholarship, and education by publishing worldwide. Oxford is a registered trade mark of Oxford University Press in the UK and certain other countries.

Published in the United States of America by Oxford University Press
198 Madison Avenue, New York, NY 10016, United States of America.

© Oxford University Press 2022

Library of Congress Cataloging-in-Publication Data
Names: Meltzer, Ethan, author.
Title: How to think like a neurologist : a case-based guide to clinical
reasoning in neurology / Ethan Meltzer.
Description: New York, NY : Oxford University Press, [2022] |
Includes bibliographical references and index.
Identifiers: LCCN 2022000243 (print) | LCCN 2022000244 (ebook) |
ISBN 9780197576663 (paperback) | ISBN 9780197576687 (epub) | ISBN 9780197576694
Subjects: MESH: Nervous System Diseases | Clinical Reasoning | Case Reports
Classification: LCC RC346 (print) | LCC RC346 (ebook) | NLM WL 140 |
DDC 616.8—dc23/eng/20220204
LC record available at https://lccn.loc.gov/2022000243
LC ebook record available at https://lccn.loc.gov/2022000244

DOI: 10.1093/med/9780197576663.001.0001

Printed by Marquis, Canada

To my father, David, for his encouragement and advice, without which this book would not have been possible.

CONTENTS

PREFACE

Given the intent of this manuscript, it is only apt that I begin with a memorable patient case.

> *The head of our department and the patient sat facing each other in amicable silence for what seemed to be 10 minutes. Neither had said a word since the department head walked into the room, introduced himself to the patient, and got only a blank stare in return. While the two looked at one another, neither apparently feeling the need to start a conversation, a whole crowd of medical students and residents watched, bewildered. As the minutes drew on, the silence grew increasingly uncomfortable. We shifted our weight from one foot to the other, and we wondered what the department head could possibly be learning about the patient from this long, awkward silence. Finally, the patient gave a large yawn. The head of the department promptly stood up, tested the patient's strength, noted subtle weakness in the patient's right arm, made some notes, and then left the room. We all followed in tow. Once we had all gathered around him, he correctly identified the diagnosis. But how?*

.

Most neurologists can remember a time early in our training when we watched with a mix of incomprehension and awe as a senior neurologist identified a mysterious affliction in a patient using just a history, his or her hands, and a collection of odd tools drawn out of an oversized bag. That I stood there slack-jawed wondering what that encounter had revealed was because at that point I had no framework or training in *clinical reasoning* in neurology.

I was hardly alone: The lack of such training is a pervasive deficit in medical education. Medical students and residents learn a very great deal about neuroanatomy, neurologic diseases, and therapeutic management. What they do *not* learn are the secrets of diagnosing neurologic disease, and the critical reasoning that underpins the process. Why? The process is rarely, if ever, expressly taught. Instead, it is perhaps assumed such skills will come with time, mentorship, and experience. They may, or they may not.

The memorable moments of the seasoned neurologist at the bedside take on mythic status. Though diagnosing a rare neurologic disease with nothing but a bedside history and exam (with perhaps a yawn for good measure) is remarkable, seeing or hearing it does not by itself lead to meaningful medical education. Trainees do not come away feeling empowered to use their own clinical judgment— since all they had done is witnessed someone else's—to come to the same conclusions. For those who do not become neurologists, the lack of clinical reasoning competency perpetuates the "black box" of neurology and leads to *neurophobia*. The veil is never lifted.

How to Think Like a Neurologist flips the neurology educational narrative on its head and attempts to lift the veil to show how neurologists use critical thinking and clinical reasoning to diagnose neurologic diseases. Although this is a case-based book, the focus is not on the diseases themselves but rather on the clinical methods used to identify neurologic diseases, and the method is disarmingly simple. The cases in this book are a fascinating collection of oddities and rarities, but the diseases themselves in this book are merely the vessel through which clinical reasoning is taught.

This book aims to provide a practical representation of the modern-day practice of medicine, where the good clinical neurologist is no longer seen as somebody who somehow carries encyclopedic knowledge of every medical condition. Rather, they appropriately recognize and categorize findings, and then, having narrowed the possibilities, they do the necessary additional research in order to appropriately diagnose and treat the patient.

ACKNOWLEDGMENTS

I would like to acknowledge Dr. Martin A. Samuels and Dr. Allan H. Ropper, who taught me how to think like a neurologist.

Initially, I gave *How to Think Like a Neurologist* as a lecture to medical students. The inspiration for this lecture, and the subsequent writing of this book, came from the teachings of Drs. Samuels and Ropper as well as from Dr. Aaron L. Berkowitz and his book, *Clinical Neurology and Neuroanatomy: A Localization-Based Approach*. I would also like to acknowledge Dr. William J. Schwartz, who encouraged me to write this book one afternoon while we were chatting in his office.

Thank you to Dr. David Paydarfar and Dr. Robin Hilsabeck for contributing several cases.

Thank you to Aaron deGruyter for providing the art found on the cover of this book.

Lastly, a special thank you to those who helped review and edit the manuscript, Dr. Kian Adabi, Dr. Zahra Cain-Akbar, Dr. Aaron Berkowitz, Dr. Amalie Chen, Dr. Amr Ellaithy, Dr. Tran Le, Dr. William Schwartz, Dr. Michael Stanley, and Dr. Joseph Yoon.

Chapter 1

How to think like a neurologist

INTRODUCTION

This will be the only chapter in this book that is not focused primarily on a case. However, this background information sets the foundation of clinical reasoning we will use for the rest of this book. The key formula and discussion is adapted and built upon from Aaron Berkowitz's *Clinical Neurology and Neuroanatomy: A Localization-Based Approach* as well as *Adams and Victor's Principles of Neurology*:

Pace + Localization = Syndrome

Syndrome + Context = Differential Diagnosis

This formula is the central guiding principle behind how a neurologist thinks. The purpose of the bedside history and examination is to define pace and localization, and all further clinical reasoning such as interpretation of laboratory values or imaging is inherently based on this foundation.

The benefits to this approach to clinical reasoning can't be overstated. Learning to use pace and localization:

- Distills the clinical syndrome to its core and allows for diagnosis of even rare disorders

- Decreases unnecessary or incorrect imaging/testing
- Prevents misattribution of imaging/laboratory findings to the patient's syndrome that might lead to misdiagnosis
- Directs the appropriate depth of the neurologic exam for that particular patient
- Helps the clinician keep track of what parts of the history and physical don't fit. As an illness evolves, these can be brought back into consideration.

You will see these benefits in the cases presented throughout the book. Learning how to utilize these formulas unlocks the ability for any individual, whether a seasoned neurologist, a medical student, or an advanced practice provider, to tackle even the most challenging cases. However, in order to utilize it in practice, we must first define and understand its terms.

WHAT IS PACE?

Pace is the onset or evolution of a patient's symptoms. You likely already incorporate many questions into your history of present illness with the intent to define the pace. When did the symptoms start? How long did the symptoms last? How have the symptoms changed since onset? Critically important in neurology, we define pace based on the initial onset and evolution of symptoms, rather than the total duration of symptoms. For example, a patient may have a fixed deficit from a stroke suffered years prior, but the pace would still be defined as quite rapid (hyperacute) if their symptoms initially developed over seconds to minutes. This principle holds true for all categories of pace.

For our discussion, we will divide pace into several broad categories, from fastest to slowest: *hyperacute, acute, subacute,* and *chronic.* The cutoffs I will use to define these categories are not formal or clearly demarcated. Although we will identify pace as fitting into one of these categories, the reality is that pace is a continuous spectrum and these categories blend into one another.

Hyperacute

Hyperacute symptoms come on over seconds to minutes. When possible, patients or their families are able to tell you exactly when and where their symptoms started. For example, you might hear from the daughter of your patient, "I was eating lunch with my mother at 1:30 when she suddenly started speaking gibberish, and her right side became weak." Alternatively, a patient might say, "I was watching television when a dark shade came over my vision. By the time the commercial break had ended, my vision had gone back to normal." When the pace is hyperacute and a history is obtainable, there is almost always a well-defined demarcation between the patient's baseline and when their symptoms started.

Of course, a clear history like those just given is not always available. In those instances (as you might encounter later in the book), the syndrome is not as easily defined, so the differential diagnosis remains broader.

Acute

Acute symptoms develop over minutes to hours to days. The boundary between the patient's baseline and the onset of symptoms is typically still clear, although there may no longer be an official "start time." For example, a friend of your patient might report, "My friend developed a fever last night. He texted me this morning that he was going to stay home from work because his head had started to hurt. When I stopped by his house this afternoon he was a little confused, but by the evening he was no longer conscious."

Subacute

Subacute symptoms develop over days to weeks to months. The boundary between the patient's baseline and the onset of symptoms starts to blur, and the patient may not be aware of when their symptoms started. However, they might remember a specific event when their symptoms first became noticeable. For example, a patient might report, "I was an avid runner, but a month ago I started noticing that it was taking me longer to do my usual route. About a week later, I tripped over a small step on the sidewalk. Since that time, I have stumbled over my left foot a few times, and my husband says that he can hear my foot dragging across our floor when I walk." Distinguishing between a subacute versus a chronic onset of symptoms might be challenging for a patient or their family (as well as the clinician) to define, since the boundary between normal and abnormal may not be clearly demarcated. Questions that attempt to draw a frame around the timeline can be helpful: "Were your symptoms present 2 months ago when you took a trip with your family?" or "When was the last time that your mother was able to handle her bills on her own?"

Chronic

Lastly, *chronic* symptoms develop over months to years. The boundary between the patient's baseline and the onset of symptoms might not exist. There is no official start time, but typically, a patient or relative can tell you a time in the patient's life when the symptoms were not present. For example, a patient's son might say, "My elderly mother has lived alone for the past several years since my father passed away. She has always been fiercely independent, and I never used to worry about her being alone. However, over the past year she is becoming more forgetful. She forgot my daughter's birthday this year, which she always celebrates by sending my daughter presents. The last time I was at her house I noticed a letter on her counter for a bill she had forgotten to pay."

Caveats

For all neurologic diseases, the pace fits into these categories. However, sometimes the pace of the underlying pathologic diagnosis is incongruent with the pace of the onset of symptoms. Take, for example, a benign brain tumor growing over a chronic time period. A patient may not develop any symptoms until the tumor causes a seizure. This would be an example of a hyperacute pace of presentation for a chronic pathology. Alternatively, a particular pathologic diagnosis might have different paces at different times. The most notorious would be the variable symptoms related to venous disease, such as venous thromboses or vascular malformations. Diseases that cause disruption in CSF flow, abnormal intracranial pressure, or other compression may have varied pace of onset. Unfortunately, there is no one-to-one correlation between syndromes and pathologic diagnoses.

Some might argue that there should be a distinct category of pace for episodic disorders (such as relapsing–remitting multiple sclerosis). My approach is to define pace for each distinct episode (which are frequently hyperacute or acute) as well as the pace of the overall course of disease. For example, a patient with no prior history of epilepsy might present with a first-time seizure. Within 2 weeks she is now having multiple seizures per day. Each discrete episode of seizure has a hyperacute onset, but the overall trajectory of her illness seems to be subacute in that her symptoms evolved over the span of several weeks. In this example, even though each seizure has a hyperacute pace, we would suspect the underlying etiology of her seizures to be a subacute process such as an inflammatory or infectious condition based on the evolution of her symptoms over several weeks.

Summary

As a rule, we can separate major etiologies of disease based on the pace of symptoms as depicted in Table 1.1.

As you can see, if we are able to clearly define the pace of the patient's symptoms, which is not always feasible in real life, we can narrow down our differential diagnosis fairly substantially to a few buckets of etiologic disease categories (with rare exceptions). This will help us take our anatomic/syndromic diagnosis and put it into a smaller pool of potential pathologic/etiologic diagnoses, as elaborated in the following sections. As mentioned previously, some etiologic diseases commonly present with multiple paces of disease. In this book, I do not focus on structural disorders, which I will define as discrete non-oncologic extra-axial compressive lesions (such as cervical stenosis or a subdural hematoma). I do not mean to trivialize these disorders. The pace of symptoms can be more highly variable. In addition, since diagnosis of these disorders tends to rely more heavily on imaging findings, I have opted to omit these from the book, which focuses more on cases where imaging might either be difficult to interpret, misleading, or unhelpful. This is an editorial choice and not because these

Table 1.1 CATEGORIES OF DISEASE BY PACE OF ONSET OF SYMPTOMS

Pace	Timing	Etiologic diagnoses	Example pathologic diagnoses
Hyperacute	Seconds to minutes	Vascular	Ischemic or hemorrhagic stroke
		Seizure	Generalized tonic-clonic seizure
		Headache	Cluster headache
		Syncope	Dysautonomia
		Trauma/structural	Fall/car accident
		Toxic/metabolic	Opiate overdose
Acute	Minutes to hours to days	Infectious	Bacterial meningitis
		Inflammatory	Optic neuritis
		Toxic/metabolic	Uremia
		Structural	Epidural hematoma
Subacute	Days to weeks to months	Infectious	Tuberculosis
		Inflammatory	Autoimmune encephalitis
		Neoplastic	Glioblastoma
		Toxic/metabolic	Vitamin deficiencies
		Structural	Subdural hematoma
Chronic	Months to years	Genetic	Huntington's disease
		Neurodegenerative	Amyotrophic lateral sclerosis
		Neoplastic	Meningioma
		Toxic/metabolic	Lead poisoning
		Structural	Cervical stenosis

disorders are not worth mentioning or commonly encountered in clinical practice.

WHAT IS LOCALIZATION?

Localization is the process of identifying "where" the lesion that causes the patient's symptoms is located in the nervous system. Again, you likely already incorporate questions in your standard patient interview that try to "localize the lesion": Where are your symptoms located? Do your symptoms radiate? Do you have any associated symptoms? These questions can help you determine, even before examining a patient, where the lesion might be located.

Localization in clinical practice

There is no shortcut to localizing the lesion. The process starts in the history, where the presence or lack of neurologic symptoms begins to narrow down what component(s) of the nervous system are involved. Many students and trainees may underestimate the role of the history in localizing the lesion. A patient who states that he initially developed painful paresthesias and numbness in his feet, and then over the next few years those symptoms slowly spread up to his knees and now involve his hands, has told you the localization (a length-dependent peripheral neuropathy). The exam that follows is done to disprove the hypothesis generated by the history. If a clinician suspects a length-dependent neuropathy, they are looking for findings on the exam that are inconsistent with that localization. Finding sensory loss as well as absent reflexes at his ankles, diminished at the patella, and present at the biceps, is simply confirmatory and does not add additional information that wasn't already available from the history. However, the presence of an unexpected finding on physical exam such as preserved or hyperactive reflexes makes the neurologist rethink the clinical syndrome.

Whether you are a seasoned neurologist or student, it is important to explicitly list the possible locations of a lesion within the nervous system. Figure 1.1 shows a schematic hierarchy and classification of localization in the nervous system. This is not intended to be an exhaustive list of localizations but rather a framework to think about the hierarchy of localization. As neurologists, we think about this at a very detailed level, and we want students and trainees to make this a habit. When localizing the lesion, start at the top and work your way down, drilling down to the most precise localization possible. Is the lesion in the central or peripheral nervous system? If peripheral, is it in the roots, plexus, nerves, neuromuscular junction, or muscle? Target your history and exam to help answer those questions, and it will make localization that much easier.

Localization takes practice and is a skill that cannot be mastered over the course of just a few weeks or even months. However, if you approach each patient attempting to "localize the lesion" in a systemic fashion, you will soon find yourself becoming more successful at making the right diagnosis and minimizing unnecessary testing.

Caveats

The lack of ability to localize a patient's symptoms to a single location in the nervous system due to either the presence of a single pathology manifesting in multiple locations, or the presence of multiple pathologies, is a common pitfall for even the most seasoned clinicians. We may initially begin this bedside exercise expecting one lesion will explain all of the patient's symptoms, but some patients will have multifocal lesions.

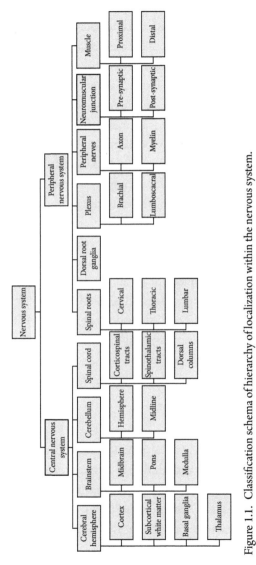

Figure 1.1. Classification schema of hierarchy of localization within the nervous system.

This is often where the *context* plays a valuable role. An 85-year-old woman with osteoarthritis, prior ischemic stroke, and diabetes who presents with difficulty walking may not have a single unifying syndrome to explain her gait difficulty. However, a 12-year-old boy who is otherwise healthy and presents with gait difficulty is unlikely to have multiple processes underlying his presentation. In general, Occam's razor, the idea that a single lesion or single pathologic process is responsible for a patient's symptoms, becomes less reliable with age. Hickam's dictum, the idea that a patient's symptoms might be due to multiple lesions or diseases, becomes more likely with advancing age.

WHAT IS THE SYNDROME?

Pace + Localization = Syndrome

In neurology, the *syndrome* is the constellation of signs and symptoms of the patient in terms of *pace* and *localization*. What we have done with this formula is to explicitly outline how to generate the "assessment" component of our encounter, which, in neurology, is chiefly composed of the clinical *syndrome*. Examples of a syndrome include rapidly progressive (acute) cervical myelopathy, or chronic (slowly progressive) length-dependent sensory and motor neuropathy.

In the cases that follow, we will define the pace of symptoms prior to discussing localization, which I have chosen to do for two reasons. First, pace is always defined during the history, whereas localization typically requires both the history and exam. At the bedside, we typically know the pace before we know the exact localization. Second, for trainees, as compared to the senior neurologist, localization can be difficult to define. Thus, pace plays a more important role in defining the syndrome. In reality, neurologists may perform a complete history and exam and then start with the localization prior to pace to help narrow down the differential etiologic diagnoses. Whether we start with pace and then go to localization or the other way around, the end result is the same: We define the clinical syndrome.

Once the syndrome is defined, then we are able to generate a differential diagnosis by adding the clinical context.

Syndrome + Context = Differential Diagnosis

WHAT IS THE CLINICAL CONTEXT?

The *context* is an independent variable of the formula, and it is chiefly derived from the history or medical record. The context, which can be relevant or irrelevant to a given presentation, is the rest of the history (medical, surgical, social, family), but it is not a product of the neurologist's analytical thinking. The context may help order the differential diagnosis, but it typically does not rule out any specific diagnosis. The differential diagnosis of a young child presenting with hyperacute loss of consciousness is ordered in a dramatically different way if the context is that she had a fall with head-strike 30 minutes prior to developing symptoms versus if the context is that she was found next to an empty pill bottle. The context is the best way to quickly narrow down the differential diagnosis, but it is also the most frequent cause of bias or anchoring. *It is critical to define the syndrome before adding the context in order to minimize the risk of anchoring.*

WHAT IS THE DIFFERENTIAL DIAGNOSIS?

What can make neurology appear so daunting to the student and neurology trainee is that the final outcome or symptom a patient reports can be attributable to numerous different anatomic diagnoses, syndromic diagnoses, etiologic diagnoses, and, finally, pathologic diagnoses. The *anatomic diagnosis* might be as simple as a patient with difficulty walking has a peroneal neuropathy. A *syndromic diagnosis* you might be familiar with would be the insidious, chronic onset of signs and symptoms of parkinsonism: moderate-amplitude low-frequency resting tremor, gait instability, rigidity, and bradykinesia. Conversely, the *etiologic diagnosis*, the mechanism of disease, for a patient presenting with sudden-onset unresponsiveness could be an ischemic infarct. The *pathologic diagnosis*, the root cause of disease, of a woman with gait difficulty might be pernicious anemia leading to B_{12} deficiency and subacute combined degeneration. Therefore, in neurology, possibly more than any other field in medicine, navigating to the right diagnosis requires the correctly sequenced approach.

Let's do a brief case to familiarize ourselves with these terms.

Case

A 50-year-old man presents to the emergency room with difficulty walking.

WHAT ARE OUR POSSIBLE ANATOMIC DIAGNOSES?

Think about the different components of the neurologic exam, which roughly correspond to different systems within the nervous system. Our patient could have trouble walking due to problems with attention or neglect (impaired mental status secondary to a non-dominant parietal lobe lesion). Our patient could have impaired walking due to a bitemporal hemianopia (cranial nerve lesion at the level of the optic chiasm). His symptoms could be the result of weakness due to an injury of the corticospinal tracts in the internal capsule, the spinal cord, the nerve roots, the neuromuscular junction, or the muscles themselves (essentially any motor lesion from the cortex all the way to the muscle). Maybe our patient has Parkinson's disease, which can cause extrapyramidal symptoms that lead to gait dysfunction ("extrapyramidal" means outside the motor tracts, such as a lesion in the basal ganglia). Perhaps our patient has loss of proprioception, which causes him to not be able to ambulate (sensory lesion). Lastly, maybe our patient has ataxia, which makes him unstable on his feet (cerebellar lesion).

As you can see, a relatively simple chief complaint can actually be quite challenging, as there can be a long list of possible *anatomic diagnoses*.

WHAT IS THE SYNDROMIC DIAGNOSIS?

Symptoms rarely exist in isolation. On top of just a single symptom of difficulty walking, our patient is likely to have other complaints. He might have pain. He could feel weak. Perhaps he is fatigued. Maybe a family member noted that he has been confused. Now, not only do we need to address and determine where his problems walking originate, but also we need to put it into context with other associated symptoms. To the trainee, this may serve to confound the question and make it more challenging to arrive at the differential. However, for the seasoned clinician, these associated symptoms can be combined to form a *syndromic diagnosis*. If our patient has hyperacute onset of difficulty walking due to right leg weakness, now we have a syndromic diagnosis that generates a limited differential of pathologic diagnoses.

WHAT IS THE PATHOLOGIC OR ETIOLOGIC DIAGNOSIS?

The *pathologic* and *etiologic diagnoses* are the final goal. For our patient who presents with hyperacute onset of difficulty walking due to right leg weakness, the *etiologic diagnosis* might be an ischemic stroke, and the *pathologic diagnosis* might be a cardioembolus from atrial fibrillation. Only after arriving at this final destination are we able to recommend appropriate treatment for the patient.

With the advent of modern imaging and other diagnostic techniques, it might seem tempting to try to leapfrog past the anatomic or syndromic diagnosis directly to the pathologic diagnosis, rather than going sequentially through the steps just laid out. Even for the seasoned neurologist, that line of thinking, in my opinion, opens the possibility for many errors—inappropriate and wasteful imaging studies, laboratory tests, delays in diagnosis and time-sensitive treatment, and incorrect diagnoses due to overreliance on ancillary data and irrelevant incidental findings. At a minimum, for you, taking these types of shortcuts actively interferes with learning.

Challenges in medical education

The typical approach to clinical cases focuses on the pathologic or etiologic diagnosis. In fact, most textbooks and standardized medical examinations, such as the shelf exam or the RITE exam in the United States, focus almost exclusively on localization or a student's ability to correctly identify the *etiologic* or *pathologic diagnoses*. However, in neurology, the challenge of an unknown case is making the connection between the localization and the underlying pathology by correctly identifying the *anatomic* or *syndromic diagnoses*. In the real world, patients do not tell you they have subacute onset

of limbic system dysfunction and then ask you to look up potential etiologies. You have to identify the *syndromic diagnosis* through
the history and physical examination at the bedside using pace and
localization. An expert neurologist (or any other physician or advanced practice provider, for that matter), excels at identifying
first the *syndromic diagnosis* from the history and physical and then
generating a list of *etiologic* or *pathologic diagnoses*. Once the appropriate syndromic diagnosis is derived from the history and physical,
the underlying etiology is then relatively easy to work up from there
with the assistance of widely available resources.

Summary

Pace + Localization = Syndrome

How does the concept of pace and localization provide a framework
for the above challenge?

Syndrome + Context = Differential Diagnosis

By identifying the onset and evolution of symptoms and where
they are located in the nervous system, we can appropriately frame
our clinical question and answer both the *anatomic* and *syndromic
diagnoses*. This framework then will allow us to formulate a differential diagnosis of the *etiologic* and *pathologic diagnoses*, which are
commonly tested for with imaging or laboratory work-up. In neurology, that may involve advanced imaging, spinal fluid analysis, or
nerve conduction studies. The challenge with the typical approach
to clinical cases is that the focus is weighted on the end result rather
than how we get there. This approach reinforces memorization of
facts, but it does not help explain the clinical method, which is how
a neurologist thinks.

Caveats

Before proceeding further, I must acknowledge that the syndromic approach is not always appropriate. In emergency situations, when a patient is critically ill or at high risk of imminent harm, we may not have the luxury of working through the clinical syndrome. We might be missing key information, or we must treat the patient for potentially reversible conditions without waiting to obtain a history (such as administering naloxone to patients who present to the emergency room in coma even if there is no confirmed history of opiate use). In addition, serious conditions with high risk of harm tend to be weighted more heavily in our differential diagnosis in emergency situations, and rightfully so. The differential diagnosis can be divided into two columns, one that encompasses the most likely diagnosis and the other that encompasses diagnoses that are "can't miss." Even if those "can't miss" diagnoses are less likely, they still must be ruled out. If we fully disregard a "can't miss" diagnosis just because it doesn't fit the framework of pace and localization, then we set ourselves up for potentially missing a critical diagnosis. Thus, in emergency situations, an algorithmic approach to generating a differential diagnosis often prevails. There is such a thing as being *too smart* in an emergency situation.

Lastly, the full syndrome may not be apparent when the patient is initially evaluated. This is particularly true for diseases with a subacute or chronic pace of disease. We may not always have the luxury of waiting for the full syndrome to develop. Alternatively, a diagnosis might not become obvious until additional symptoms develop. In this sense, any case-based exercise that presents a syndrome that spans a prolonged time period is artificial. In the real world, we often must act before having all the information at hand.

ORGANIZATION OF THE REMAINING CHAPTERS

The remainder of this text will focus on case presentations. You will be given a history and examination, and we will work through each case together, defining both the pace and localization. From there, we will define the syndrome, and, at times utilizing the context, the ultimate etiologic and pathologic diagnoses. The goal is to learn the process, which is how a neurologist thinks. I will provide the end diagnosis and a brief discussion of the pathologic diagnosis for each case. However, the focus of the cases is on the process, *not* on the diseases themselves.

The cases will be roughly ordered by escalating complexity. The titles of each case are intentionally vague, so as not to reveal the diagnosis. In addition, they are not ordered by pace, localization, or etiology so as not to be predictable.

When you hear hoof beats, think of horses before zebras. If you have not heard this adage before, it means that the symptoms of a patient can be attributable to many different diagnoses. However, common diseases are common, and rare diseases are rare. A skilled clinician will always incorporate the pre-test probability of a given disease when generating a differential diagnosis. His or her differential is not a laundry list of highly unlikely rare disorders; rather, each potential disorder is weighted by its prevalence in the population and context. However, for the remainder of this book, you will only encounter zebras and, occasionally, a horse that is masquerading as a zebra. These cases will almost exclusively cover rare diseases you may have never heard of or cases that are highly atypical presentations of more common diseases.

The purpose of only using zebras is two-fold. First, it will remove all risk in participating. Using only rare cases removes some of the desire to skip to the end to read the answer after the case is presented. Yes, the answer will be at the end, but I can promise you that you are very unlikely to know it based on reading just the first few lines of the case presentation. You can take a shortcut, but you will not be rewarded with having "guessed it right" based on the information given in the first few sentences of each case. The only way to learn from each case is to work through the thought exercises. This book is about the process or journey to the diagnosis, not the diagnoses themselves. I strongly advise you not to use this book to learn about specific diseases processes; there are many other resources out there already for that purpose, which I mentioned earlier.

The second purpose of using zebras is much simpler. One of the unique aspects of neurology compared to other medical specialties is the sheer breadth of pathophysiology and different presentations of disease. Zebras are fascinating, and neurology has the best zebras in all of medicine, although I might be a bit biased. Others seem to agree—that is the reason why the "Case Records of the Massachusetts General Hospital" published in the *New England Journal of Medicine* is disproportionately composed of neurologic cases. It is the same reason medical TV shows such as *House* also feature so many neurologic diseases.

I recommend that you attempt to work through the cases as you read. The book is best enjoyed interactively. I encourage you to use any references you would like as you work through the cases. Most of the cases require a basic understanding of neuroanatomy that is covered in medical school, and I include relevant neuroanatomy diagrams when I am able. However, you might find it helpful to refer to diagrams about neuroanatomic pathways while you read each case. Looking something up isn't cheating.

The practice of medicine allows you to utilize any resources you desire.

Lastly, the case vignettes I present are all real patients. The history, examination, and data presented are all real, although minor components of the history may have been altered to obscure identifying details.

Chapter 2

A woman with rapid onset of aphasia

Let's go through this case together to get you acclimated to the exercise of identifying *pace* and *localization*. This one is a warm-up we will do together to introduce you to the framework of the rest of the book.

A 32-year-old right-handed woman at 33 weeks gestation presented to the hospital with confusion and altered speech. She initially developed diffuse headache as well as neck pain on the day of presentation. Approximately 2 hours after onset of headache, she noted sudden onset of decreased sensation over her right arm. She also developed difficulty speaking, which she described as being able to think of a word but having a difficult time saying it. She had an MRI of her brain that was unremarkable and was admitted to the hospital for observation. Her pregnancy had been unremarkable to date with the exception of an upper respiratory tract infection earlier in the month. After her upper respiratory tract infection resolved, she was treated with amoxicillin for otitis media in the days leading up to her presentation.

The remainder of the cases in this book will follow the same format. Typically, I will try to include any relevant past medical history or other context that was available at the time. The histories are abbreviated, and you may not receive the full history that was collected at the time of the encounter for the sake of brevity. However, I will not hide relevant information from you that was available at the time of evaluation. Prior to presenting the exam, I will bring up key points to consider. In these cases, just as in real life, the exam occurs after the history. Work along at home while you read the history and exam. Think about what questions you would have asked or what you would have tested on exam.

She became increasingly agitated and combative over the next several hours after admission. On repeat examination, she was no longer verbal and could no longer follow commands. Shortly thereafter, she became comatose and was intubated. No reliable neurologic exam was able to be performed at that time due to the sedating medications she was given during intubation. Although initially afebrile on presentation, she eventually spiked a temperature to 102.2°F.

WHAT IS THE PACE?

First, we need to define the rapidity of the onset of her symptoms. Time zero is the onset of her first neurologic symptoms. In this case, it is when she developed a headache. From there, she had progressively worsening symptoms over the span of several hours that culminated in coma. The time from onset of symptoms to intubation was hours. Return to the categories of pace defined in Chapter 1 if needed. Which category does this fall into? Was the onset of her symptoms hyperacute (seconds to minutes), acute (hours to days), subacute (days to weeks), or chronic (months to years)?

Based on these definitions, we can classify the pace of her symptoms as acute. In addition to this acute pace, her course was also punctuated by more sudden onset of decreased sensation over her right arm and speech difficulties. This is consistent with an overlapping hyperacute onset of new symptoms that might allude to a somewhat distinct process. Although we could start generating a differential diagnosis of various potential etiologies of her presentation, I urge you to work through this example in a stepwise fashion for learning purposes. Let's now tackle the localization.

WHAT IS THE LOCALIZATION?

Even without having a reliable neurologic exam, we can localize the lesion based on her history. What are the key aspects of the history that will help us localize the lesion?

- Headache and neck pain
- Language dysfunction
- Decreased sensation of her right arm
- Decreased consciousness

We can approximate the localization of her lesion using these components of the history. Headache and neck pain indicates a process that involves the head or neck. Next, her language dysfunction can be characterized as a non-fluent aphasia. She described it as being able to think of the appropriate word but not being able to produce language. This would localize to Broca's area, found in the frontal lobe of the dominant hemisphere. For a right-handed individual (and a large percentage of left-handed individuals), this is the left frontal lobe. Decreased sensation of her right arm could localize to anywhere from the sensory strip located along the left post-central gyrus of the lateral parietal lobe down to the peripheral nerves. However, if her symptoms are due to one lesion rather than multifocal lesions (not always the case), then her sensory dysfunction likely localizes to the left parietal lobe.

Lastly, she eventually had decreased levels of consciousness. Briefly, coma implies that as her disease progressed, she had more widespread involvement of the brain. The localization of coma will be expanded upon in later cases. Taken together, the initial localization of her symptoms is the left frontal and parietal lobes, with spread over hours to more global cerebral dysfunction.

Now that we have identified the pace and localization, we can define the clinical syndrome.

Pace + Localization = Syndrome

WHAT IS THE SYNDROMIC DIAGNOSIS?

She presents with acute onset of an initially left frontal and parietal lobe syndrome that progresses to generalized cerebral dysfunction. The differential diagnosis of categories of disease with a pace that is acute is relatively short: infectious, inflammatory, and toxic/metabolic disorders.

WHAT IS THE ETIOLOGIC DIAGNOSIS?

Only now, after defining her clinical syndrome, we will add the context to generate our differential diagnosis.

Syndrome + Context = Differential Diagnosis

For her case, the context is key. The top of our differential diagnosis must be infectious etiologies. She is a young woman with a recent history of otitis media who now presents with headache, neck pain, and acutely-evolving loss of consciousness with high fevers. The context in this case screams "infection." Her presentation is concerning for bacterial meningitis secondary to her otitis media. Although in this case the context was paramount in coming to the correct diagnosis, in the remaining cases in the book, just as in the real world, the context may not be as helpful or might even be misleading. Before proceeding to the final pathologic diagnosis and conclusion of the case, let's see how her clinical course progressed.

CLINICAL COURSE AND ADDITIONAL INFORMATION

Her cerebrospinal fluid was markedly abnormal. The opening pressure was 50 cm H_2O (normal 10–25). Cerebrospinal fluid showed 3,710 WBCs/μL (normal <5), total protein of 192 mg/dL (normal 15–45), and a glucose of 1 mg/dL (normal 40–70). Cerebrospinal fluid cultures grew *Streptococcus pneumoniae*.

She dramatically improved with treatment over the next 24 hours to the degree that she was successfully extubated. Although she was no longer comatose, she had persistent neurologic dysfunction. She was now awake, alert, and oriented, but she could not follow 2-step commands. She was able to name objects, and she could repeat. Her speech was effortful, and she spoke in short phrases. When presented with a complex picture, instead of describing the entire scene together, she could only describe small parts of the scene at any given time (simultanagnosia). She had a mild hemiparesis of her right upper and lower extremities. She had decreased sensation on her right side.

How do we explain her focal deficits: non-fluent aphasia, simultanagnosia, and right upper extremity motor and sensory symptoms? Now that we can get a more detailed exam, it is worth going back to localization before we conclude.

WHAT IS THE LOCALIZATION?

Her exam is notable for persistent focal deficits that we have not yet been able to explain. She now has a new deficit, simultanagnosia. This is the inability to comprehend a complex visual depiction despite the retained ability to identify individual details. Simultanagnosia is likely due to a deficit in sustained attention to visuospatial information and the synthesis of visual information. It localizes to the

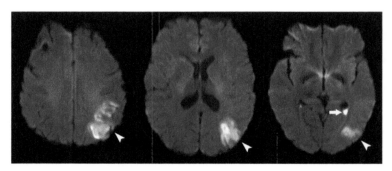

Figure 2.1. MRI brain axial DWI sequence. The three *arrow heads* point to an area of hyperintensity in the left frontal, parietal, and occipital lobes, which is consistent with acute infarction in the territory of her left middle cerebral artery. The *arrow* denotes an area of increased signal in her ventricles consistent with ventriculitis.

inferolateral part of the dominant parieto-occipital lobes. This new deficit again points us to a cortical process involving her dominant (left) frontal, parietal, and now occipital cortices. Why might a woman with meningitis have a persistent focal deficit? Her initial MRI brain was normal, but given her persistent deficits, a repeat MRI brain was obtained.

We have now identified the etiology of her hyperacute (sudden) onset of sensory and language dysfunction. Her MRI brain shows an acute ischemic infarct (Figure 2.1).

CONCLUSION

The final pathologic diagnosis for this case was bacterial meningitis due to *Streptococcus pneumonia* due to contiguous spread from otitis media complicated by secondary acute ischemic stroke in the territory of her left middle cerebral artery. Bacterial meningitis can result in acute ischemic stroke, and the proposed mechanism is likely direct endothelial damage and inflammation secondary to bacterial infection. She went on to make a full neurologic recovery, and she gave birth to a healthy baby girl at term.

Chapter 3

A woman with sudden numbness

A 60-year-old right-handed woman presented with numbness. She was sitting at her office at work when she suddenly developed numbness over her entire right leg. She denied any pain or paresthesias. She described the numbness as involving her entire right leg from her foot to her waistline. Over the next few minutes, her symptoms spread to involve her buttocks, the right side of her torso, and the lateral aspect of her right arm. Two hours after her symptom onset, she described feeling "odd" and "a little fuzzy in my head." She denied any other associated neurologic or systemic symptoms, including no confusion, changes in vision, difficulty speaking, weakness, or bowel/bladder dysfunction.

Sometimes the exam I present is a basic screening neurologic exam. Other times the exam I present will include additional exam maneuvers. In these cases, part of the learning is from thinking about why that specific exam was performed. Based on this history above, what components of the screening neurologic exam might you expand upon?

On examination, she had mild hypertension with a blood pressure of 148/92. She was well-appearing. Her mental status was normal, and there were no cranial nerve abnormalities. Muscle bulk and tone were normal. Her strength was normal, including no pronator drift. She had decreased sensation to light touch, vibration, and pinprick circumferentially around her right lower extremity, abdomen and chest up to approximately T6, and over her right arm. Her reflexes were normal, and her toes were down-going bilaterally. She had no dysmetria, and her stance and stride were normal.

Although in most cases I won't provide you with any data prior to working through the pace and localization, in this case I will provide the initial MRI results.

She had an MRI brain and spine that was interpreted as having no evidence of stroke, hemorrhage, tumor, or other explanation for her symptoms.

WHAT IS THE PACE?

The pace is all about the very beginning of the onset of symptoms. She provides an excellent history that her symptoms evolved over seconds to minutes. That is consistent with a pace that is *hyperacute.*

WHAT IS THE LOCALIZATION?

She presents with isolated sensory symptoms and signs on examination. This is truly a pure sensory syndrome. The fact that everything else is completely normal is quite helpful in localizing the lesion. We know that the lesion must be isolated to the ascending sensory pathways, and it must be in a place where it can cause profound sensory deficits while somehow leaving other neurologic function intact. Both the medial lemniscal pathway and the spinothalamic tract originate from the periphery and terminate in the sensory cortex. Please reference Figure 3.1 for a depiction of these ascending somatosensory pathways. However, the critical question is where along these pathways is the lesion. The pattern of her sensory dysfunction seen on her examination can help us narrow down the potential localizations.

Could the lesion be located in the peripheral nervous system?

Given the lack of motor involvement, the lesion can't be in the muscles or at the neuromuscular junction. Theoretically, it could involve just the sensory components of the peripheral nerves, roots, or dorsal root ganglia. However, multiple parts of the peripheral nervous system would have to be involved instantaneously through multiple different simultaneous lesions, which seems unlikely. Here, the hyperacute pace actually helps us to rule out the peripheral nervous system as a potential etiology. A peripheral neuropathy can arise acutely from ischemia (such as in vasculitis), but it seems incredibly unlikely that she would develop simultaneous isolated sensory deficits throughout the right side of her body due to damage of the peripheral nerves. Thus, it is unlikely for the lesion to fall within the sensory pathways in the peripheral nervous system.

Where in the central nervous system is the lesion?

Let's start from the bottom of the spinal cord and work our way up. She has sensory deficits involving the right upper extremity, torso, and right lower extremity. Since the arm is involved, the lesion must be above the thoracic spine, as the sensory fibers from the upper

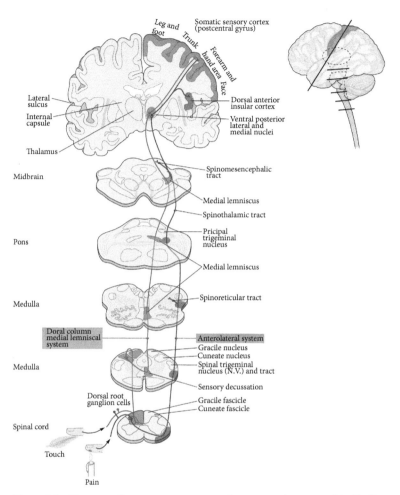

Figure 3.1. The ascending somatosensory pathways remain geographically distinct throughout the spinal cord and brainstem until the level of the midbrain. Until these pathways converge, a single lesion involving both the spinothalamic tract and medial lemniscus would be sufficiently large to cause other neurologic deficits. *Republished with permission of McGraw Hill LLC, from* Principles of Neural Science, *Kandel, Eric R., James H. Schwartz, Thomas M. Jessell, Steven A. Siegelbaum, and A.J. Hudspeth, 5th edition, 2012; permission conveyed through Copyright Clearance Center, Inc.*

extremities enter in the cervical cord. In addition, she has deficits attributable to both the spinothalamic tract and the dorsal column on the same side. However, the spinothalamic tract is crossed in the spinal cord, but the dorsal column is uncrossed. Thus, her syndrome would require two lesions in the spinal cord or a single large lesion involving both sides. Given the lack of any other symptoms of a myelopathy such as weakness or bowel/bladder dysfunction, a large spinal cord lesion is unlikely.

We run into a similar problem in the brainstem that we encountered in the spinal cord. Although the fibers from the medial lemniscus cross in the medulla and are on the same side as the spinothalamic tract rostral to that decussation, they ascend the brainstem more medially compared to the ascending fibers of the spinothalamic tract. For much of the brainstem, until the midbrain when the fibers start to come together, we would likely need a large lesion. In a large brainstem lesion, we would expect to see deficits in cranial nerves, which are not present on exam. Figure 3.1 depicts the relationship of the ascending somatosensory pathways in the brainstem.

By process of elimination, we are left with the lesion being somewhere in the brain. I know many of you had already honed in on the brain, especially given her history of "feeling off" and "fuzzy" in her head. Where in the brain is the lesion? We are searching for a place where all the sensory fibers are together in close proximity where a small lesion can cause profound sensory loss but somehow avoid causing any other neurologic deficit (or be readily apparent on imaging). As the tracts ascend through the brainstem they finally merge together and synapse in the ventral posterior lateral nucleus of the thalamus. From there, they make their final ascent together through the posterior limb of the internal capsule prior to reaching the primary somatosensory cortex, where they fan out over a large area. The only place along the sensory tracts where we can get isolated sensory loss of multiple modalities due to a very small lesion that might not be apparent on imaging without other neurologic deficits is in the thalamus or ascending third-order neurons prior to the cortex. It is in these locations that the fibers occupy a very small space and damage can cause an isolated sensory syndrome. We now have our localization.

WHAT IS THE SYNDROMIC DIAGNOSIS?

She presents with hyperacute onset of sensory loss due to a lesion in either the ventral posterior lateral nucleus of the thalamus or internal capsule. That is her *syndromic diagnosis*.

WHAT IS THE ETIOLOGIC DIAGNOSIS?

Now that we have defined her syndromic diagnosis, let's determine the *etiologic diagnosis*. Because her syndrome presented hyperacutely, we know that the underlying etiology is likely to be due to either a vascular process or a seizure. Although a traumatic injury or toxic process is possible, there is no supporting *context* for either of these etiologies. Seizure is a possible explanation to her presentation, but given the lack of a classic seizure syndrome, and the fact that she now has fixed deficits that are absence of function (negative rather than positive symptoms), it is also less likely. Thus, we are left with a vascular etiology as the most likely cause of her presentation.

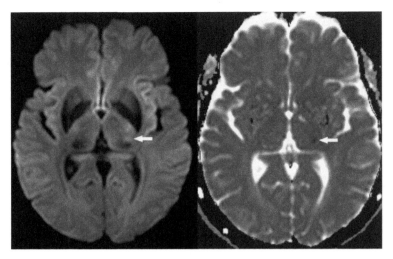

Figure 3.2. MRI axial brain DWI (*left*) and ADC (*right*). The *arrows* point to the small areas of hyperintensity on the DWI sequence and hypointensity on the ADC sequence consistent with acute infarction.

CONCLUSION

Let's take another look at the MRI brain that was obtained and initially interpreted as normal.

Upon further review of her MRI depicted in Figure 3.2, there is a small, but definite, area of restricted diffusion abutting the ventral posterolateral nucleus of the left thalamus consistent with an acute lacunar infarction. The most likely etiology of her stroke was small vessel disease. This is a great example of the fact that an image that is obtained for a patient is only as good as the history and exam. Without the information gleaned from the bedside, a crucial diagnosis would have been missed.

Chapter 4

A woman who couldn't hold a cigarette in her mouth

A 49-year-old right-handed woman with a history of smoking and alcohol use disorder presented with difficulty speaking and swallowing. She initially noticed that she would occasionally cough after eating or drinking. She also noted that her voice was less clear than normal. Unfortunately, her symptoms worsened over the next year. She could no longer close her lips tightly together to hold a cigarette in her mouth. She began using her fingers to move food toward the middle of her mouth to help her swallow. She carried around a notebook to write everything down, as she was no longer able to speak, although her writing was fluent, and she had no difficulty with comprehension. Approximately 1 year after her initial symptoms, she developed weakness in her right arm and leg. She noticed that the muscles of her right leg appeared smaller than the left. She had difficulty flexing at the ankles in both feet, which resulted in frequent falls. She denied any vision changes, headache, tremor, or sensory changes.

Just as in our first examples, let's pause after the history before we move on to the exam. There is a lot that is abnormal in her history, and I am sure that many of you already have diagnoses that are jumping into mind. However, the point of this book is to learn to think like a neurologist. That means that we cannot simply jump to a list of diseases.

When I hear this history, the first thing I think about is: What is the cranial nerve exam? I suspect that there will be abnormalities related to strength of the face and oropharynx. However, are there abnormalities of her extraocular muscles? That might change my localization. Likewise, I suspect I will encounter weakness with strength testing, but what pattern will I see? Will she have sensory deficits? What will the reflexes show? These are the questions that will help us more definitively localize the lesion. The exam is not just about finding a sign that matches a symptom a patient reports. We will use the exam to confirm or refute our hypothesized localization.

Her mental status was normal. She was unable to phonate and could only make guttural noises, but she was able to communicate by writing. Her vision and extraocular movements were normal. She could not purse her lips together or puff out her cheeks. Her tongue had decreased bulk. Fasciculations were present in her tongue and masseters. She was unable to push her tongue into her cheeks. She had decreased muscle bulk in the right thigh and leg. She had fasciculations in her deltoids and quadriceps bilaterally. Strength testing revealed scattered weakness (ranging MRC grade 4– to 4+) involving right shoulder abduction, the intrinsic muscles of her right hand, right hip flexion, right knee flexion/extension, and right ankle plantar flexion. She had severe weakness with dorsiflexion bilaterally (1 on the right and 3 on the left). Her reflexes were brisk, including the presence of a glabellar reflex, jaw jerk, Hoffman's sign, and Babinski's sign. The sensory and cerebellar examination was normal. She had a steppage gait.

WHAT IS THE PACE?

Her symptoms appear to have evolved over the past year (at least). She doesn't report a specific day she noted her symptoms beginning; rather, the onset is insidious. She then has definite worsening that takes place over the next months to year. This is all consistent with a pace that is *chronic*.

WHAT IS THE LOCALIZATION?

We have a lot to think about with her history and her exam. There is no single way to organize the approach to localization. For this case, I will go through her symptoms in chronological order to help us organize our thinking.

Her initial symptoms are that of dysarthria and dysphagia. These symptoms have several different possible localizations. They could be the result of an injury to the cerebral hemispheres, such as in a stroke. They could be due to a lesion in the brainstem involving the various cranial nerve nuclei responsible for coordinating the muscles of the pharynx. There could be a cerebellar lesion. Alternatively, a disorder of the nerves themselves could cause these symptoms. These symptoms could easily arise from a problem at the muscle or even neuromuscular junction. As you can see, a single symptom in and of itself may not be helpful. This is where the exam comes into play.

We see evidence of severe weakness of the mouth, tongue, and lower face on exam, but that was expected based on her history. What other features of her exam help us to narrow down the localization? We don't see evidence of any other cranial nerve dysfunction besides the muscles involving the mouth and lower face. That makes a more widespread brainstem process unlikely. In addition, we see fasciculations of the tongue. What does that tell us? We see fasciculations when there is a visible contraction of a muscle fascicle. These are the result of spontaneous and sporadic discharges of dysfunctional lower motor nerves. This is a very helpful observation: We now know that whatever the underlying pathology, the lower motor nerves are affected.

Although her symptoms were initially isolated above her neck, over time she developed involvement of her arms and legs. We might ask ourselves: What is the pattern of weakness of her extremities? The pattern is that there is no pattern. It doesn't follow a gradient such as proximal more involved than distal. Both sides are involved. Not all muscle groups are affected equally. This lack of pattern, the fact that it involves both upper and lower extremities bilaterally to various degrees, can be helpful. That seems less consistent with a myopathy (these often have a pattern of weakness such as a proximal to distal gradient), and it is less consistent with a brain/spinal cord lesion given the sporadic nature of her deficits. We again see fasciculations, which, as we mentioned earlier, indicate the lower motor nerves are involved. Decreased muscle bulk is also consistent with a lower motor nerve process.

Now, let's discuss the rest of her exam.

Her sensory exam is entirely normal. We know that her lower motor nerves are involved, but with normal sensation, this cannot be a generalized peripheral neuropathy. If that were the case, she would have both motor and sensory loss.

She has strikingly brisk and pathologic reflexes. What might you expect her reflexes to be (increased or diminished) if this

Table 4.1 COMPARISON OF SYMPTOMS DUE TO AN UPPER VERSUS
LOWER MOTOR NEURON LESION

	Upper motor neuron	Lower motor neuron
Tone	Increased	Decreased
Muscles involved	Always in groups	Can be individual muscles
Fasciculations	Absent	Can be present
Reflexes	Hyperactive and pathologic	Diminished or absent
Electrophysiology studies	Normal	Abnormal

were a pure lower motor nerve process? This cannot be due to an isolated peripheral nervous system disease and the lower motor neurons alone as that would cause diminished or absent reflexes— the corticospinal tracts must be involved. Thus, we know that the upper motor neurons must be involved as well as the lower motor neurons. Please see Table 4.1 for common signs of upper and lower motor neuron dysfunction.

We have enough to put this case together.

WHAT IS THE SYNDROMIC DIAGNOSIS?

She presents with chronic onset of signs and symptoms that localize to an upper and lower motor neuron disease.

WHAT IS THE ETIOLOGIC DIAGNOSIS?

The most likely potential etiologic diagnoses include neurodegenerative and genetic causes of upper and lower motor neuron dysfunction. Other etiologies such as toxic or metabolic etiologies are less likely given the lack of context in her history.

CONCLUSION

Unfortunately, the list of possible pathologic diagnoses for chronic onset of upper and lower motor neuron disease is short. Many of you may have already guessed the pathologic diagnosis purely based on her history. However, this case was relatively straightforward, and it is only a warm-up for the more esoteric cases to come.

The most common cause of progressive upper and lower motor neuron dysfunction is amyotrophic lateral sclerosis (ALS). ALS is one of a family of neurodegenerative disorders that primarily affects the motor neurons. Some of these disorders predominantly involve the lower motor neurons (progressive muscular atrophy), some predominantly involve the upper motor neurons (primary lateral sclerosis), and some involve both upper and lower motor neurons (ALS). The clinical evolution is variable. In our case, she had bulbar-onset ALS with later spread to her limbs. Unfortunately, her condition progressed, and she ultimately passed away from ALS within a year of her diagnosis.

Chapter 5

A woman who didn't realize she couldn't see half the world

A 43-year-old woman went to her optometrist for a routine eye appointment. The patient noted no visual disturbances, such as blurred or decreased visual acuity, double vision, enlarged blind spots, or change in color vision. Her medical history was significant for diabetes, hypertension, and glaucoma. However, these were well controlled, and she did not have diabetic retinopathy or glaucoma-related optic neuropathy. Her optometrist noted the patient had a visual field cut, so she referred her to the emergency room for urgent neurology evaluation. The patient denied any headaches, confusion, changes in her speech, weakness, changes in sensation, or urinary dysfunction. Even after being told by her optometrist about this abnormality in her vision, the patient was unaware of any abnormality with her vision unless she specifically tested it.

In this case, the patient was unaware of any deficit. This can be a clue to the pace, but it can also make the localization challenging. We cannot tailor her examination based on her history as we would normally like to do. Because of her lack of symptoms, we will need to perform a very careful screening neurologic exam.

On examination, her mental status was normal. Cranial nerve examination was notable for normal visual acuity bilaterally. Funduscopic exam revealed sharp optic discs bilaterally without evidence of papilledema. She had loss of the temporal visual field of her left eye and the nasal visual field of her right eye. Her pupils were equal and reactive to light. Color vision was normal. The rest of her neurologic exam was normal, including strength to confrontation testing, sensation, reflexes, and gait.

WHAT IS THE PACE?

This one is a bit tricky, since there is not much of a clinical history provided. However, that same lack of history can serve as our biggest clue as to the pace of disease. What is the most likely time course of the onset of her symptoms that would make such a severe deficit imperceptible to the patient? If we approach the problem this way it starts to become clear that whatever the cause of her symptoms is, it likely didn't come on suddenly. To have such a noticeable deficit on exam the patient was unaware of and to not have *any* other abnormalities on her neurologic exam or symptoms, it likely came on slowly over time. Compensation requires time, so this must be a very slow-moving, chronic process.

WHAT IS THE LOCALIZATION?

She has loss of the temporal visual field on one side and the nasal visual field on the other. Both hemi-field losses are occurring on the left side of the visual world. The terminology used to describe this neurologic deficit is a left homonymous hemianopia. Since we are neurologists, let's take this one step farther and ask where along the anterior visual system a lesion can cause a homonymous hemianopia.

A homonymous hemianopia is a field defect involving half the visual field, and it is homonymous when they are located similarly in the visual fields of both eyes. These lesions occur at the level of or after the optic chiasm, often referred to as retrochiasmal. There are additional subtleties and associated clinical findings that can help to further localize the lesion; however, those are beyond the scope or intent of this book. The key take-home for the localization here is that a homonymous hemianopia simply tells us the lesion is retrochiasmal. It does not further localize, without associated features or more in-depth examination, whether the lesion is found in the optic tracts, optic radiations, thalamus (lateral geniculate body), or occipital lobes. Please see Figure 5.1 for a depiction of the various deficits that can arise from lesions along the visual pathways from the optic nerves to the primary visual cortex. And for those of you guessing at potential etiologic diagnoses, the finding of a homonymous hemianopia is certainly not always a posterior cerebral artery stroke.

ADDITIONAL INFORMATION

Figure 5.2 depicts several representative images of an MRI of her brain obtained at the time of her presentation. The findings are not subtle. How do we reconcile this striking image with her relatively normal neurologic exam and the fact that she is unaware of her deficits? If you took a guess or two at diagnoses that is okay—but

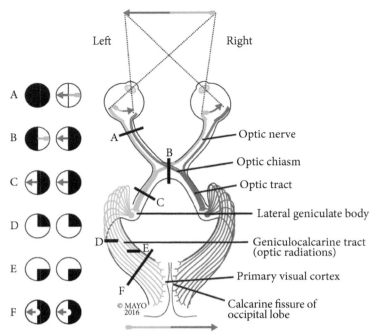

Left   Right

A

B — Optic nerve

— Optic chiasm

C — Optic tract

— Lateral geniculate body

D — Geniculocalcarine tract (optic radiations)

E — Primary visual cortex

F — Calcarine fissure of occipital lobe

© MAYO 2016

Figure 5.1. The visual field deficit is dependent on the location of the lesion along the visual pathways. Retrochiasmal lesions (examples C–F) can cause a homonymous deficit. The degree of visual field loss depends on the location and size of the lesion. *Reproduced by permission from Benarroch, Eduardo E., Jeremy K. Cutsforth-Gregory, and Kelly D. Flemming, Mayo Clinic Medical Neurosciences: Organized by Neurologic System and Level (New York, New York: Oxford University Press, 2017).*

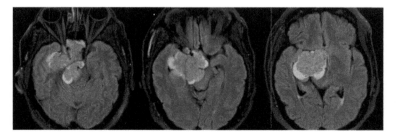

Figure 5.2. MRI axial brain FLAIR sequence. There is a large lesion with irregular borders involving the brainstem, thalamus, and other deep gray nuclei on the right side.

remember, that is not the purpose of the book. Don't worry, we will make a diagnosis, but we aren't there quite yet. This is about the process, not the final outcome. Let's go back to the basics.

WHAT IS THE SYNDROMIC DIAGNOSIS?

This is a 43-year-old woman who presents with a slowly progressive, chronic lesion in her brain causing an isolated left homonymous hemianopia.

WHAT IS THE ETIOLOGIC DIAGNOSIS?

Our possible *etiologic diagnoses* consist only of very slowly evolving intracranial processes. Thus, even though you may not be familiar with interpreting brain MRIs, you can reasonably exclude hyperacute and acute processes such as strokes or hemorrhages. These diseases could not present with so few symptoms, as their pace of onset is too fast to allow for any sort of compensation. In fact, the degree of mass effect involving the deep structures of the brain and brainstem, if secondary to a hemorrhage, would almost certainly be fatal. Likewise, other faster and more destructive processes such as infections or malignant tumors are highly unlikely due to the relative normalcy of her presentation.

Of the etiologic diagnoses that cause chronic disease, we can throw out neurodegenerative diseases, as those shouldn't cause a large intracranial lesion. We can also remove congenital and genetic syndromes for the same reason, and because these would also be less likely to present this late in adulthood with a focal mass.

We are left with benign intracranial tumors as the only cause of a chronic, slow-growing intracranial lesion that is not causing overt signs of tissue destruction. At this point our etiologic diagnosis has been whittled down to a single category of disease. Although it might not seem like it at first, we have actually gotten almost as far as we need to (or can) without getting a biopsy to make a pathologic diagnosis.

For those of you who want to go a step further and name the tumor, keep reading along.

CONCLUSION

Although the list of benign intracranial tumors involves some rare entities found in reference textbooks, there are a handful of common tumors that you are likely to encounter. These include meningiomas, the most common benign intracranial tumor in adults; schwannomas (sometimes referred to as acoustic neuromas if they involve the vestibulocochlear nerve); low-grade gliomas; and pituitary adenomas.

Notice that I have been using the term "intracranial." We can further localize whether our lesion is inside the brain parenchyma or outside the brain parenchyma, referred to as *intra-axial* or *extra-axial*, respectively. Take a closer look at the MRI. Is the image intra-axial or extra-axial?

The lesion is extra-axial. If you look closely, you can see that it is displacing the brain, not infiltrating it. Our short differential diagnosis gets shorter. Ultimately, the diagnosis was made in the operating room. She had a pituitary macroadenoma, but can we predict whether it was secreting or non-secreting?

This was a non-secreting pituitary macroadenoma, which is what allowed it to grow relatively asymptomatically for many years without her noticing. If this had been a secreting pituitary adenoma, she likely would have developed symptoms (such as galactorrhea) long before it reached this size.

Unfortunately, although she was found to have a benign tumor, the surgery and subsequent management was complicated due to the size of the tumor and its close proximity and encroachment on many critical structures.

Chapter 6

A woman who developed weakness after windsurfing

A 27-year-old woman went windsurfing while on vacation with her family. At the end of the day her neck felt stiff, so she intentionally "cracked" it by quickly rotating it to one side. She immediately developed weakness in her bilateral upper extremities to the point that she was unable to lift her arms off her bed. Within a few hours of onset of her symptoms she had difficulty ambulating. She developed urinary retention with no sensation of bladder fullness. This was so severe that she had over a liter of urine in her bladder that drained after a Foley catheter was placed.

Before you read further, pause and start to form a hypothesis about what the exam might reveal. The history is not just about identifying the pace, but it is the start of localization. Based on the history, do you suspect this is a lesion involving the central or peripheral nervous system? If you suspect a lesion in the CNS, where might it be and what findings (present or absent) might support your hypothesis? If you suspect a lesion in the PNS, what might be different? As you read the exam below, remember that our exam is informed by the history. Try to take a minute before proceeding to think about what exam maneuvers you might include (or exclude) when examining the patient.

Her neurologic examination was notable for normal mental status and cranial nerves. Her strength was 0/5 in the bilateral proximal upper extremities (shoulder abduction, elbow flexion and extension). Her strength was 3 to 4–/5 in the distal upper extremities (wrist flexion and extension, intrinsic muscles of the hand). Her strength in the proximal lower extremities was 3 to 4–/5 (hip flexion, knee flexion and extension), and her strength was normal in the distal lower extremities. She had completely absent sensation to pinprick and temperature below her neck; however, she had preserved sensation to vibration and position. Her reflexes were diminished throughout, and her plantar response was "mute."

She was initially seen at an outside hospital where she had an MRI of her brain and spine, which were normal. Due to the diagnostic uncertainty of her presentation, she was transferred to our facility for a second opinion.

WHAT IS THE PACE?

Although her symptoms continued to progress over several hours after initial onset, the symptom onset was quite rapid over seconds to minutes, which fits with a hyperacute time course of disease.

WHAT IS THE LOCALIZATION?

First, we must decide whether her symptoms are attributable to a lesion in the central or peripheral nervous system. She has dissociated loss of pinprick and temperature with preservation of vibratory and position sense. Remember, these fibers travel together in the periphery via peripheral nerves to the dorsal root ganglia. Once these fibers enter the spinal cord, they split into the spinothalamic tracts (pain and temperature) and dorsal columns (vibration, proprioception, fine touch, and two-point discrimination). The spinothalamic tracts synapse and decussate soon after entering the spinal cord and ascend in the anterolateral cord, whereas the dorsal columns synapse in the dorsal root ganglia but do not decussate until they reach the medulla via the posterior cord (Figure 6.1). Since our patient has dissociation of sensory modalities, we know that the lesion cannot be in the peripheral nervous system and must be central. The dissociation of sensory modalities also localizes within the central nervous system to the spinal cord given her lack of cranial nerve abnormalities. Even though these pathways remain separate in the lower brainstem, making the brainstem a theoretical localization (see Chapter 3, Figure 3.1), the fact that her deficits are all below the neck strongly indicates the lesion is within the spinal cord.

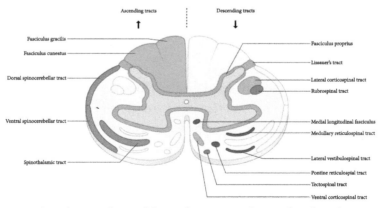

Figure 6.1. The ascending and descending tracts in the spinal cord are shown in cross-section. Note the locations of the fasciculus gracilis and cuneatus (dorsal column), lateral corticospinal tract, and spinothalamic tracts. *This figure was published in Neuroanatomy: an Illustrated Colour Text, 6th edition, Alan R. Crossman and David Neary, Page 77, Copyright Elsevier (2019).*

Let's follow Occam's razor and see if we can identify one spinal cord lesion that can cause all of her symptoms. Of course, this is not always true, and a patient can have multiple lesions. She is weak bilaterally, so we know that both corticospinal tracts are involved. Given the predominant involvement of the upper extremities more so than the lower extremities, we might suspect a central cord syndrome. This is because the corticospinal tracts are organized somatotopically, with information traveling to the upper extremities found medially and information to the lower extremities traveling laterally. Usually in a central cord syndrome, the sensory deficit is a cape-like decrease of pain and temperature. This arises from dysfunction of the crossing spinothalamic fibers in the anterior white commissure at the level of the lesion. The spinothalamic fibers from levels more caudal to the lesion are only involved in much larger lesions, as they are found more laterally in the spinothalamic tract.

However, our patient has profound and complete loss of sensation to pain and temperature. This implicates a much larger lesion than just the central cord that extends to cover both spinothalamic tracts and most of the corticospinal tracts (medial more than lateral). The lesion would therefore need to cover most of the anterior spinal cord, but it must spare the posterior cord since vibration and position sense traveling in the dorsal columns are preserved.

Lastly, we know that the lesion must be in the cervical spinal cord, since it involves myotomes and dermatomes in the upper extremities.

WHAT IS THE SYNDROMIC DIAGNOSIS?

Our patient is a 27-year-old woman who presents with a syndromic diagnosis of hyperacute onset of an anterior spinal cord syndrome.

WHAT IS THE ETIOLOGIC DIAGNOSIS?

The etiologic differential diagnosis for hyperacute neurologic syndromes in this case is essentially limited to either trauma or a vascular event. She has a history of neck manipulation (clinical context), which raises the question of a traumatic lesion. However, the initial MRI of her spine did not show any abnormalities. We would expect to see pathologies causing a compressive myelopathy, such as an epidural hematoma or ruptured disc, to be present on her MRI. Since those are absent, then a vascular etiology becomes the most likely cause of her neurologic deficits.

This is where our knowledge of neuroanatomy is once again important. Since we suspect a vascular event, we need to know the vascular supply to the spinal cord. The anterior spinal cord is perfused by the anterior spinal artery, which originates from the two vertebral arteries. Several small branches contribute to it along its course running down the spinal cord, the largest of which is named the artery of Adamkiewicz and typically originates in the lower thoracic cord. The anterior spinal artery perfuses the anterior two-thirds of the spinal cord, and the posterior spinal artery perfuses the posterior one-third of the spinal cord. The posterior spinal artery resembles more of an anastomotic network of small vessels rather than a single, dominant vessel like the anterior spinal artery. Because of that, it is much less at risk of hypoperfusion or infarct.

The territory of the spinal cord supplied by the anterior spinal artery includes both the corticospinal tracts and the spinothalamic tracts but spares the dorsal columns. Thus, our patient's *anatomic diagnosis* is consistent with an anterior spinal artery syndrome, and her syndromic diagnosis with hyperacute onset of symptoms points to a vascular event. Armed with the knowledge of her exam, we repeated an MRI of her cervical spine, this time with a sequence to look for stroke. This MRI confirmed the suspected *etiologic diagnosis*. She had suffered an infarct of her anterior spinal artery.

Without the formulation of our syndromic diagnosis, we never would have obtained the MRI shown in Figure 6.2. This is a sagittal ADC sequence of the cervical spine, which is not part of a typical spine MRI protocol. The arrows on the image show the area of signal hypointensity present in the anterior cervical cord spanning

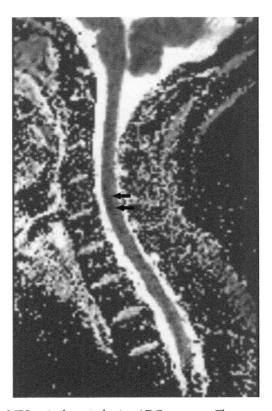

Figure 6.2. MRI sagittal cervical spine ADC sequence. The *arrows* point to an area of signal hypointensity within the anterior cervical cord consistent with acute infarction.

C4–C5. This is the area of infarct. Note that the posterior spinal cord at that level is normal. Although the MRI is quite striking, it was merely confirmatory for a diagnosis that was made at the bedside.

CONCLUSION

The suspected *pathologic diagnosis* of her infarct was a fibrocartilaginous embolism. The proposed mechanism is that a small embolus of material from an intervertebral disc caused by minor trauma travels through one of the smaller arteries feeding the anterior spinal artery. This embolism then becomes lodged in one of the distal branches of the anterior spinal artery that perfuses the spinal cord, leading to infarction. Since the posterior spinal artery perfuses the posterior third of the spinal cord, that part of the spinal cord is unaffected. This is a rare condition, and certain individuals might be at higher risk due to persistent intervertebral vasculature that typically involutes during development or revascularization during normal aging. Treatment is typically supportive, although some institutions will place a lumbar drain to decrease intracranial pressure by draining off CSF in an attempt to maximize perfusion pressure and increase blood flow.

Ultimately, she recovered full strength in her right arm and lower extremities. However, her left arm remained weak. She had persistent severe neuropathic pain as well as bowel and bladder dysfunction. This degree of motor recovery is expected based on her score on the ASIA (American Spinal Injury Association) Impairment Scale, which is a standardized exam to assess motor and sensory dysfunction after spinal cord injury. This scale can be used to predict long-term recovery of neurologic function.

Chapter 7

A man who became unresponsive

A 61-year-old man with a past medical history of atrial fibrilla-tion presented with abrupt onset of coma. He was in the kitchen washing dishes with his wife when he suddenly exclaimed, "Oh God, I don't feel right." His wife asked what was wrong, and he replied that he felt dizzy and that he couldn't see. He walked over to a couch to lie down, and within a minute he was unrespon-sive. He was in a deep coma when the paramedics arrived several minutes later, and he needed to be intubated in the emergency room as he was having difficulty breathing on his own. His wife denied any suspicion for substance abuse or toxic ingestion. There was no history of trauma.

This is a highly concerning history. As discussed in the introduc-tion, the algorithmic approach to management in this case is appro-priate and what the emergency medicine physicians pursued. They went down a list of "can't miss" diagnoses: hypoglycemia, drug over-dose, etc. However, they were also the ones who obtained the exam (detailed next) when something seemed "off." Even in emergency settings, non-neurologists can utilize the framework of pace and lo-calization to appropriately diagnose and treat a patient.

On arrival to the emergency room, his vitals were stable. His eyes were closed, and he was unresponsive to noxious stimuli.

His right pupil was minimally reactive and larger than the left (anisocoria). He made no spontaneous purposeful movements, and he exhibited decorticate posturing.

He had no abnormality on labs obtained in the emergency room, including electrolytes, kidney and liver function, and toxicology screening. He had a CT as well as a CT angiogram of his head and neck; results were normal. There was no evidence of hemorrhage, tumor, or stroke on his CT, and his angiogram did not show any thromboses. At that point, the emergency room physicians contacted neurology for evaluation. Despite the normal head imaging, they were still concerned for a primary neurologic process based on their exam findings. By the time neurology arrived, no repeat exam could be performed as he had recently received sedation during his emergent intubation to help protect his airway due to persistent coma.

WHAT IS THE PACE?

This patient presents with evolution of symptoms over seconds to minutes, which fits with a hyperacute time course of disease.

WHAT IS THE LOCALIZATION?

Even though we can't perform a detailed neurologic examination, we can use his history and the limited exam provided to localize the lesion.

What is the localization of impaired consciousness?

Of course, this localizes to the central nervous system. However, we can take an even more detailed look at *where* consciousness is derived from within the central nervous system. The ascending arousal system receives both excitatory and inhibitory from many aspects of the nervous system to regulate normal sleep and wake cycles. The key components involve the reticular formation in the upper brainstem (mid-pons and above), thalamus, hypothalamus, basal forebrain, and cortex (Figure 7.1). Thus, a lesion in any of these locations has the potential to depress consciousness. Given the widespread network involved in regulating consciousness, lesions

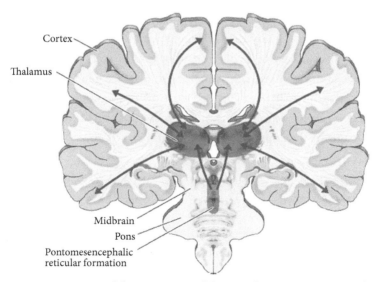

Figure 7.1. Drawing of the projections of the reticular activating system. The reticular formation in the upper brainstem radiates widely to other parts of the brain, including the thalamus and cortex. *Reproduced by permission from Hal Blumenfeld, Neuroanatomy through Clinical Cases (New York, New York: Oxford University Press, 2018), 41.*

must be bilateral to cause sufficient disruption in this network to cause coma. Lesions that are unilateral are (typically) not sufficient to cause impaired arousal on their own—for example, a large left middle cerebral artery stroke may cause hemiplegia and mutism, but it will not cause coma (unless through a secondary means such as mass effect on the contralateral hemisphere or brainstem).

Once we identify what structures must be involved in coma, then we can start to localize the lesion. We are essentially left with a lesion involving the bilateral cerebral hemispheres, thalami, hypothalamus, or paramedian brainstem rostral to the mid-pons. Impaired arousal is, unfortunately, commonly seen in the emergency room and in the hospital. In these settings, it is very commonly due to bilateral cortical injury. Even though you may not have thought about consciousness this way previously, you likely have seen this localization play out many times. Patients who present with decreased arousal secondary to alcohol or other toxic ingestion, severe metabolic abnormalities such as hyponatremia, or a generalized tonic-clonic seizure all have bilateral cortical dysfunction. You might be less familiar with lesions or disorders that might preferentially damage the thalamus, hypothalamus, or brainstem.

What other clues in the history and examination can help us to further localize the lesion?

He noted dizziness and vision impairment prior to slipping into coma. In addition, his examination revealed decreased pupil reactivity and anisocoria. Although we can't ask him further questions to elaborate on what he meant by the word dizzy (imbalance, vertigo, light-headedness), the presence of dizziness accompanied by vision changes and ocular findings is suspicious for cranial nerve dysfunction and a brainstem process. More specifically, the pupillary light reflex pathway involves afferent fibers traveling from the retina through the optic nerve to the pretectal nucleus in the midbrain. That signal is then transmitted back to the eye via the efferent pathway from the Edinger-Westphal nuclei to the ciliary ganglion via the parasympathetic fibers in cranial nerve III.

His pupil abnormalities, reported history of dizziness (possibly vertigo), and coma can all be localized to the upper brainstem or thalamus. However, we did not see any abnormalities on his head CT. What is our next step?

WHAT IS THE SYNDROMIC DIAGNOSIS?

He has hyperacute onset of a suspected upper brainstem/thalamic injury.

WHAT IS THE ETIOLOGIC DIAGNOSIS?

Let's put everything together. Our differential of etiologic diagnoses for hyperacute processes is fairly limited. We have ruled out metabolic as well as toxic causes of his presentation, and his history doesn't note any trauma. We are essentially left with either seizure or vascular disorders. Although seizure is possible, he has not had any witnessed seizure activity (although seizures can be non-convulsive and impair consciousness), and he has some focal findings on exam that localize to the brainstem. Seizures arise from the cortex, so they should not cause findings that localize to the brainstem. At this point, even though his initial imaging was negative, a vascular cause of his presentation (ischemic stroke), is still the most likely etiologic diagnosis.

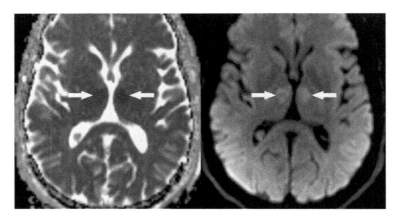

Figure 7.2. MRI axial DWI and ADC sequences at the level of the thalamus. The *arrows* point to areas of increased signal on DWI and decreased signal on ADC consistent with acute infarction.

Now that we have our etiologic diagnosis set, we can take a look at an MRI of his brain, which was obtained emergently (Figure 7.2).

His MRI shows an area of restricted diffusion in the medial and anterior bilateral thalami. In addition, his infarct involved the paramedian midbrain (not pictured). These findings can fully explain his presentation. He has injury to his bilateral thalami as well as the paramedian midbrain, which are both critical components of the ascending arousal system.

CONCLUSION

How does he have such an extensive infarct without any evidence of a blood clot on his CT angiogram? In this particular case, he had a rare anatomic variation of the perfusion of the thalamus and the midbrain. He had a small, single artery called the artery of Percheron that perfused this very large vascular territory, which is typically perfused by more than one vessel. He was unfortunate to have had a small blood clot travel up and lodge precisely in this single small arterial branch of the basilar artery (not visible on CT angiography), which caused a stroke in his midbrain and both thalami.

You might be wondering why this matters. This is a rare anatomic variant presenting with a rare stroke syndrome. However, he received treatment with tPA prior to the MRI confirming the stroke based purely on the pace and localization of his presentation. If the emergency room physicians hadn't used the principles of pace and localization, he would have been unlikely to receive treatment emergently, which likely saved his life.

Chapter 8

A woman who appeared intoxicated

A 28-year-old woman with a history of metastatic Merkel cell carcinoma of the left parotid gland presented with imbalance and visual disturbance.

She initially noted onset of imbalance while walking down a hill on a hike with her family. She felt off balance and tripped, which was unusual for her. She realized that she was having difficulty fixating her eyes on the ground in front of her, and she had the perception that the ground was moving, even if she was standing still. There was no directionality to this perception of environmental movement, and it was present in primary gaze as well as if she looked in any direction. Within a few days of symptom onset, her condition had worsened to the point that she could no longer text or use her phone because her eyes couldn't focus on the screen. She worked as a hairdresser, and she had no difficulty manipulating scissors or a comb. However, she was told not to come to work because her coworkers and clients thought that she had been drinking when they observed how unstable she was on her feet. She could easily write with a pen, but she frequently wrote letters on top of one another because she couldn't determine their precise location on the page due to the near-constant perception of environmental movement. Within a week of onset of symptoms, she could no longer walk without assistance, and she had several falls. She denied any dysarthria, dysphagia, weakness, or numbness. She was on no new medications, and she did not take any drugs or supplements. She denied any recent illnesses.

Imbalance is one of the most common chief complaints in neurology, and it can be one of the most challenging. For the patient, imbalance is what might concern them the most, but for the neurologist, imbalance is a common end result for a variety of neurologic insults. There are numerous potential localizations to a chief complaint of imbalance that can localize from the cortex (with etiologies as obscure as neglect from nondominant parietal lobe dysfunction) all the way down to the toes (due to peripheral nervous system dysfunction such as neuropathy or myopathy). The key to localizing imbalance is to try to identify the specific neurologic system(s) that are responsible for the patient's symptoms. Thus, the neurologic exam should be tailored to these entities. Is there a visual disturbance? Is it vestibular? Cerebellar? Extrapyramidal? Motor? Sensory? Based on this patient's history, where might you expect the lesion? Let this guide your exam.

On examination, her mental status was normal. She had direction-changing nystagmus during the encounter in both primary and all directions of gaze. She had hypermetric and hypometric saccades. Motor, sensory, and reflex testing were normal. She had no dysmetria with finger-to-nose, and she had no tremor. She was unable to stand with her feet together or apart without assistance. She had severe gait ataxia, and she was unable to walk without maximal assistance.

WHAT IS THE PACE?

She presents with onset of symptoms that evolved over the span of several days, which fits with an acute time course of disease.

WHAT IS THE LOCALIZATION?

Her examination is notable for severe gait ataxia as well as severe, direction-changing nystagmus. What can we glean from her findings that help us to localize the lesion? As opposed to nystagmus of vestibular (peripheral) origin that is unidirectional and increases in intensity when the eyes look in the direction of the fast phase, nystagmus of cerebellar (central) origin frequently changes direction with the direction of gaze. Thus, her direction-changing nystagmus on exam must localize to a "central" cause. Typically we think of central nystagmus and other signs of oculovestibular incoordination as originating from the cerebellum, specifically the vermis or flocculonodular lobe (Figure 8.1).

In addition to her nystagmus, she had severe truncal ataxia. She was unable to stand with her feet together or apart due to disequilibrium. Her gait was also markedly ataxic. Perhaps surprisingly, she had a remarkable lack of limb ataxia. In fact, she was so unaffected, she was still able to cut her clients' hair, a testament to the divided functions of the cerebellum (see Figure 8.1). Anatomically, the cerebellum is divided into three parts: the flocculonodular lobe, the anterior lobe, and the posterior lobe. However, the physiologic functions of the cerebellum seem to be divided from midline radiating outwards. Whereas lesions of the cerebellar hemispheres (lateral) cause incoordination of the ipsilateral limbs, lesions of the midline vermis typically lead to dysfunction in stance and gait.

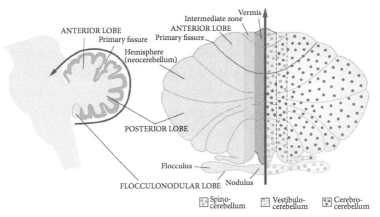

Figure 8.1. Functional organization of the cerebellum. Lesions of the cerebellum cause various syndromes depending on their location; midline lesions tend to cause truncal ataxia due to disruption of spino-cerebellar connections, hemispheric lesions tend to cause appendicular ataxia due to disruptions of cerebro-cerebellar connections, and lesions of the flocculonodular lobe or vermis tend to cause oculovestibular incoordination due to disruption of vestibulo-cerebellar connections. *Reproduced by permission from Per Brodal, The Central Nervous System Structure and Function (New York, New York: Oxford University Press, 2004).*

Occasionally, ataxia can be caused by severe loss of sensation (proprioception). When ataxia is due to loss of proprioception, then postural instability is uncovered when the patient loses visual input (such as when they close their eyes). This is not the case here: She is unstable with her eyes open and feet together and feet apart, which indicates cerebellar rather than proprioceptive dysfunction. In addition, she has normal sensation and reflexes, which makes a peripheral neuropathy unlikely.

Therefore, we predict a cerebellar lesion involving the vermis and/or flocculonodular lobe with sparing of the cerebellar hemispheres.

WHAT IS THE SYNDROMIC DIAGNOSIS?

If we combine the pace and localization, then her *syndromic diagnosis* is an acute onset of a midline (vermian and/or flocculonodular) cerebellar syndrome. Given the preservation of limb coordination, we would expect the cerebellar hemispheres to be unaffected.

WHAT IS THE ETIOLOGIC DIAGNOSIS?

The acute onset of her symptoms helps us narrow down the most likely etiologic diagnoses to include infectious, inflammatory, and toxic disorders. Although mass lesions could theoretically cause these symptoms (such as an infratentorial tumor or other cause of extrinsic compression), the rapidity of onset of her symptoms is quite striking and likely too fast to be due to even the fastest-growing tumors. In addition, the lack of other signs or symptoms, such as brainstem dysfunction or cerebellar hemispheric dysfunction, is notable. We might expect that if her symptoms were caused by something exerting mass effect evolving that rapidly, such as a hemorrhage within a tumor causing rapid expansion, she might have other abnormalities on her neurologic exam, such as signs and symptoms of brainstem compression.

At this point, the *context* comes into play. Of the most likely *etiologic* diagnoses, most involve laboratory testing. Plenty of toxins can cause an acute cerebellar syndrome, alcohol being the most common offending agent. However, other prescription medications and environmental toxins can also cause similar symptoms. The same holds true for infectious cerebellitis, which is associated with numerous (typically viral) infections. Infectious cerebellitis can be either the result of direct infection or a post-infectious (inflammatory) disorder. There was no history of medication use or toxic ingestion, and she had no recent illnesses, making infectious or toxic etiologies of her symptoms unlikely. However, her medical history was notable for Merkel cell carcinoma. How might this be related?

CONCLUSION

Her initial imaging and laboratory work-up, including an MRI of her brain and basic cerebrospinal fluid studies, was normal.

Take a moment before going forward and type the following into your favorite search engine:

Rapidly progressive cerebellar ataxia

Odds are that you will find paraneoplastic or autoimmune cerebellar degeneration within the top few hits. The suspicion for an autoimmune cerebellar syndrome (and in her case paraneoplastic, given her recent diagnosis of cancer) was quite high. She was empirically treated with intravenous immunoglobulins for a presumptive pathologic diagnosis of paraneoplastic cerebellar degeneration. Eventually, antibodies to the P/Q-type calcium channel were found in her spinal fluid, confirming the diagnosis. With prompt treatment, she made a full neurologic recovery.

Chapter 9

A man who appeared jumpy

A 71-year-old man with a history of type 2 diabetes mellitus developed abnormal movements in his right arm and leg. Four days prior to presenting to the hospital he noted onset of abnormal twitching and movements in his right arm and leg. He couldn't remember whether the movements were present on awakening that day or if his symptoms progressed during the day. Since he noticed them, the intensity of the movements remained static and isolated only to the right side. The movements were nearly continuous while he was awake, but he said if he concentrated he could make them temporarily abate. His family said the movements disappeared when he was asleep. When he walked he appeared "jumpy," but he had not fallen. He was right-handed, and he had difficulty using utensils and buttoning his clothes. Outside of these movements he otherwise felt well. He denied any headache, weakness, or sensory changes. He and his family did not think he had experienced any decline in cognition. Initially, he wasn't particularly concerned, but when his symptoms weren't improving, his family convinced him to come to the hospital for evaluation.

Frequently, the exact pace of the patient's symptoms is unclear. When that is the case, you might not be able to precisely nail down the pace, but you can still set an upper or lower bound of the timeline to help narrow down the syndromic diagnosis. Remember, pace refers to the rapidity of the onset of symptoms as well as how they change over time. If two patients wake up with the same set of symptoms, but in one scenario those symptoms worsen over the course of the week but the other patient's symptoms don't further worsen, that can be a major clue to the pace and the underlying etiology.

On examination, his mental status was normal. He was mildly anxious, but well-appearing. His cranial nerves were normal. He exhibited near-continuous uncontrollable, arrhythmic, jerking movements of his right arm and leg. In the proximal arm and leg these movements were higher amplitude than in the distal extremities, where the movements were lower amplitude. If he concentrated, he could incorporate some of these movements into more purposeful actions. Although he could briefly suppress the movements, they inevitably returned during the examination. The left side was unaffected. His strength on confrontational testing was full. He had normal sensation, and his reflexes were normal. His gait had a "dance-like" or, as his family described, "jumpy" quality to it—he seemed to incorporate these involuntary movements into his stride.

WHAT IS THE PACE?

In this case we don't have a precise timeline of symptom onset. It is possible that he awoke with these symptoms, in which case the onset could have been over seconds, minutes, or hours while he was sleeping (hyperacute or acute). Alternatively, his symptoms

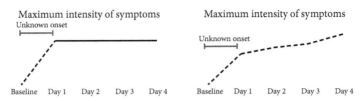

Figure 9.1. Hypothetical pace of symptoms with unknown onset. A hyperacute or acute onset of symptoms (**left**) might be more likely to be static after the initial injury, whereas an acute to subacute process (**right**) might continue to worsen after the initial unknown onset.

could have arisen over the course of the first day. If that were the case, the onset is more likely to be acute rather than hyperacute. In either scenario, we can identify an upper bound of the pace of onset.

Even though we do not know the exact timeline of the onset of symptoms, we know that the symptoms, once noticed, did not continue to worsen in intensity over the next several days. He had brief periods of time where he could consciously suppress the symptoms or they would abate during sleep. The fact that the intensity of his symptoms remained static after initial onset points toward a hyperacute or acute process that "completed" its onset during that unknown time window rather than an acute to subacute process that started during the unknown time window but continued to progress. This concept is depicted in Figure 9.1.

WHAT IS THE LOCALIZATION?

Unlike in some of the other cases we have already reviewed, there isn't much doubt that the lesion is in the central nervous system. The examination described earlier is notable for a striking unilateral hyperkinetic movement disorder. These "extrapyramidal symptoms" point the finger squarely at the basal ganglia. However, since we want to think like neurologists, let's get more specific.

We now know that the basal ganglia are responsible for multiple parallel circuits modulating eye movements, cognition, and emotion in addition to motor function. However, for the purposes of this discussion, we will focus purely on their role in the control of motor activities. The basal ganglia comprises the caudate nucleus, putamen, globus pallidus, subthalamic nucleus, and substantia nigra. The caudate and putamen are essentially continuous with each other and are referred to as the striatum. The basal ganglia exerts its influence on the cortex via the ventrolateral and ventroanterior nuclei of the thalamus.

Undoubtedly you have seen, likely several times, complex diagrams like the one depicted in Figure 9.2 showing the various inhibitory and excitatory connections between the earlier-listed nuclei within the basal ganglia that make up the motor circuit. The role of the basal ganglia in modulating motor activity can be distilled into two pathways. The *direct* pathway serves as a "switch" to activate a certain motor program (such as throwing a ball). The *indirect* pathway serves as a "brake" to prevent unwanted motor activity. Neurologic symptoms arise when the relative contributions of these pathways are imbalanced. Increased contribution of the indirect pathway over the direct pathway leads to a loss of the ability to initiate movement, causing hypokinetic movement disorders. Conversely, increased contribution of the direct pathway over the indirect pathway leads to a removal of motor inhibition and hyperkinetic movement disorders. In this case, the patient has involuntary movements that best fit the description of chorea/ballismus, implicating a lesion that causes a relative increase in contribution of the direct over the indirect pathway. Thus, the lesion could cause his

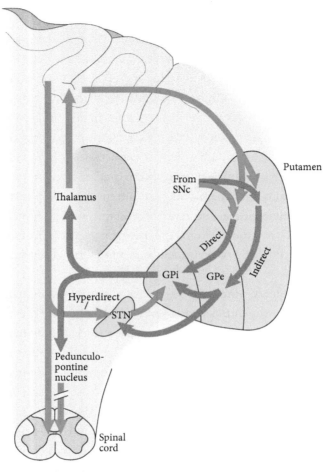

Figure 9.2. Basal ganglia.

A simplified diagram of the direct and indirect pathways of the basal ganglia. *Pink arrows* indicate activation and *blue arrows* indicate inhibition. The net effect of the direct pathway activates thalamocortical projections, whereas the net effect of the indirect pathway inhibits thalamocortical projections. Abbreviations in figure: SNc—substantia nigra pars compacta, GPi—globus pallidus internus, GPe—globus pallidus externus, STN—subthalamic nucleus. *Republished with permission of McGraw Hill LLC, from Principles of Neural Science, Kandel, Eric R., James H. Schwartz, Thomas M. Jessell, Steven A. Siegelbaum, and A.J. Hudspeth, 5th edition, 2012; permission conveyed through Copyright Clearance Center, Inc.*

symptoms through either increased activity of the direct pathway or decreased activity of the indirect pathway.

WHAT IS THE SYNDROMIC DIAGNOSIS?

Let's first put together the pace and localization. The *syndromic diagnosis* is either a hyperacute or acute illness that localizes to the basal ganglia leading to relative dysfunction of the indirect pathway compared to the direct pathway.

WHAT IS THE ETIOLOGIC DIAGNOSIS?

The pace helps us to narrow down our differential diagnosis substantially. The disorders you might typically associate with chorea or ballismus, such as Huntington's and other neurodegenerative processes, are ruled out by the rapidity of onset of his symptoms. A slow-growing or even fast-growing tumor is also unlikely to cause such abrupt onset of symptoms.

The list of most likely *etiologic diagnoses* includes vascular, infectious, or inflammatory disorders in addition to toxic or metabolic disorders. The *context* of the case helps to narrow down the differential diagnosis further. There is no indication he has a systemic infection (such as influenza, which can lead to chorea due to an encephalitis), nor is there anything in the history to suggest a systemic autoimmune disease that could lead to various neurologic manifestations. An autoimmune etiology is possible, such as a paraneoplastic syndrome. However, the pace even for an autoimmune disease is likely too fast, and left untreated, we might expect continued worsening rather than a plateau in severity of his symptoms. Thus, we are left with the *etiologic diagnosis* most likely being of vascular etiology or the result of a toxic/metabolic process.

CONCLUSION

Ultimately, imaging of his brain did not show any abnormalities in the basal ganglia, which ruled out vascular etiologies (ischemic and hemorrhagic stroke) as the cause of his presentation. The only remaining potential etiology was a toxin or metabolic derangement. His initial blood glucose on admission was 453 mg/dL (normal less than 100 mg/dL if fasting). Given the lack of structural causes evident on imaging, the working *pathologic diagnosis* was hyperglycemic, nonketotic hemichorea/hemiballism (diabetic striatopathy). This is a rare manifestation of hyperglycemia that typically presents with hemichorea/hemiballism with or without associated imaging abnormalities in the striatum. His symptoms fully resolved with insulin and intravenous hydration, which clinched the pathologic diagnosis. Further work-up for alternative non-structural causes of acute-onset hemichorea/hemiballism (such as autoimmune or paraneoplastic etiologies) was not pursued since his symptoms rapidly resolved with treatment.

Chapter 10

A woman who only ate fast food

A 37-year-old woman developed abnormal behaviors. She worked as a schoolteacher and lived at home with her husband and daughters. The first change in behavior her family noticed was she began obsessively purchasing expensive concert tickets and following a particular band touring across the country. Around this time, she also became more withdrawn from her husband and developed outbursts of anger. The following year she developed numerous obsessive behaviors, such as repeatedly locking and unlocking doors. She also began to discuss her bathroom habits with others. She stopped cooking and only ate limited items from fast-food restaurants, which led to a 30-lb weight gain. Two years after symptom onset, she began to make inappropriate sexual comments to others. Her family took away her car after they observed she would become disoriented in familiar places. Three years into her symptoms, she was no longer working due to several incidents of inappropriate behavior at work. Her husband stopped traveling for work so that he could assist her at home due to her engaging in dangerous behaviors such as "playing" with the gas stove.

This is one of those instances in which a rich history is as good as an exam. The family's observations of her behavior over years provide better insight into her condition and deficits than any brief exam performed in the clinic. I include her examination next, as well as neuropsychological testing, for the sake of completeness. The purpose of the exam is to formally assess which cognitive domains are most affected.

On examination, she was cooperative, but at times she demonstrated inappropriate laughing and smiling that was incongruent to the situation. She had minimal insight into her behaviors. She stood and walked around the clinic room, and she repetitively punched her fists together and scratched her fingernails. She scored 27/30 on the MMSE (recall was 0/3). The rest of her neurologic exam was unremarkable. She subsequently underwent neuropsychological evaluation, which revealed significant deficits in the domain of executive functioning.

WHAT IS THE PACE?

She presents with symptoms that evolved over months to years, which is consistent with a chronic pace of illness.

WHAT IS THE LOCALIZATION?

What are the salient features of her history and exam, both what impairments are significant and what are lacking? As discussed in Chapter 16, the components of the mental status that are normal are often just as important at helping localize the lesion as the components that are abnormal.

Her initial symptoms include inappropriate/disinhibited behaviors. She made expensive purchases that were uncharacteristic for her. This progressed to abnormal compulsive behaviors and situationally inappropriate and childlike behavior. Behavioral changes can occur in many different neurologic diseases but most commonly are related to dysfunction of the frontal lobes.

Lesions to the frontal lobes can result in numerous abnormalities, such as motor dysfunction, incontinence, gait abnormality, apathy/ akinesia, and personality changes, among other symptoms. Many of these symptoms are poorly localized to one specific area within the frontal lobes, which are likely involved at a high level of regulating many cognitive functions. We commonly refer to this role of the frontal lobe as *executive function*.

Executive function is what allows us to learn and adapt our behaviors based on our environment and past experiences to accomplish the task at hand. When this is disrupted, a patient frequently loses the ability to accomplish the complex tasks associated with daily life and is no longer able to live independently. Depending on the location of frontal lobe disruption, there might be various cognitive or behavioral changes associated with executive dysfunction.

There are overlapping syndromes of behavioral abnormalities associated with frontal lobe lesions, such as abulia or akinetic mutism versus the hyperactive and compulsive behaviors that our patient exhibited. Instead of being withdrawn from the outside world, she seems unable to navigate it appropriately. She has lost her sense of social cues, and her behaviors seem to be primarily motivated by personal gratification. A discussion about the specific networks within the frontal lobes is beyond the scope of this book. However, this syndrome of disinhibited, socially inappropriate behavior and executive dysfunction most likely localizes to the medial-orbital parts of the frontal lobes.

Although she does have impaired recall on examination, her history, and neurologic impairment, is clearly driven primarily by her change in personality and abnormal behaviors, rather than an amnestic syndrome. In many neurodegenerative processes, the order of onset of symptoms is important. For example, a patient with dementia that precedes the development of parkinsonism might be diagnosed with Lewy body dementia, whereas a patient who initially develops parkinsonism followed years later by cognitive impairment likely has Parkinson's disease. Individuals with Alzheimer's disease frequently develop changes in personality and behavior, but those changes typically occur later in the illness secondary to more global cognitive impairment. The fact that her changes in personality and behavior were her initial dominant symptoms out of proportion to other cognitive dysfunction helps us to localize the lesion to a frontal lobe process.

WHAT IS THE SYNDROMIC DIAGNOSIS?

She presents with a syndromic diagnosis of chronic onset of frontal lobe dysfunction.

WHAT IS THE ETIOLOGIC DIAGNOSIS?

Many neurologic disorders might begin with what is initially perceived by the patient, the patient's family, and healthcare providers as a psychiatric rather than a neurologic illness. This is one of the more common diagnostic errors made by clinicians. This is where pace and localization play a vital role. Often it simply takes time for an illness to "declare itself" and for the diagnosis to become apparent. This requires patience on the part of the clinician and careful explanation to the patient or their family that it might take time (months or even years) to make an accurate diagnosis.

Since her dysfunction is localized to the frontal lobes, it seems less likely that this could be the result of a toxic or metabolic process, which we might expect to cause more global cortical dysfunction. A slow-growing tumor or other mass-occupying lesion (such as a large frontal meningioma or subdural hematoma) could cause her symptoms. However, an MRI of her brain did not show any compressive lesions. Thus, we are left with an *etiologic diagnosis* of a neurodegenerative/genetic illness. Of those categories, is there one that fits her syndrome?

CONCLUSION

She was given the diagnosis of probable behavioral-variant frontotemporal lobar degeneration (bvFTLD), which is a collection of *pathologic diagnoses* that selectively involve the frontal and temporal lobes to varying degrees. Of note, there are other clinical presentations of FTLD due to the predominant location of pathology within the frontal and temporal lobes. Histopathology studies typically show accumulation of either tau or TDP-43 inclusions. However, there are other rarer pathologic variants. I fear making a comment that will be obsolete at the time this case is being read in the future, but at least at present, distinguishing between these various pathologic subtypes of bvFTLD is challenging in the absence of a biopsy or autopsy. Unfortunately, at present, treatment is limited and identification of the specific pathology causing the clinical syndrome is of research rather than clinical use.

Chapter 11

A woman whose cruise
was cut short

A 70-year-old woman presented with several weeks of numbness over her left upper back and abdomen. She described her initial symptoms as true loss of sensation as well as paresthesias over her left upper back and abdomen. She initially attributed her symptoms to shingles, which she had experienced several years prior. She then went on a cruise to the Caribbean; however, her symptoms progressed to a band of numbness from her umbilicus to her groin. She also noted that her left leg was numb to the touch.

She left the cruise early after she developed weakness in her left leg, which made it difficult for her to climb stairs. This was accompanied by paresthesias along the medial aspects of both arms to the fifth digits as well as hyperesthesia of the right leg.

Besides the prior episode of shingles, her past medical history was otherwise only notable for hypertension, which was well controlled on medication. She denied any prior neurologic symptoms except for the episode of shingles, and she denied any recent or remote trauma.

One of the most important decisions a neurologist makes is what parts of the neurologic exam to perform. There are situations in which the basic "screening" exam is insufficient to appropriately localize the lesion. When a patient gives a history that suggests a particular localization, like in this case, we should adapt our exam based on what the patient reports. Based on the history just provided, what is your initial hypothesis of the localization and what aspects of the neurologic exam would you focus on? What features would you test on exam in a more in-depth fashion than what you might typically do for a more basic screening exam?

If you don't know the answer to that question, that is okay. Read the following exam and think about why certain components were tested.

On examination, her mental status and cranial nerve testing was normal. Motor testing in the upper extremities and the right lower extremity was normal. Her left lower extremity was weak, 4 to 4– throughout, including a left foot drop. Sensory testing revealed decreased pinprick sensation in the right lower extremity below the waist. She had absent vibratory sensation in the left leg at the toes, medial malleolus, patella, and iliac crest. She also had patchy sensory loss to light touch over the back and abdomen. The plantar response of the right toe was down-going and the left toe was up-going. She had no axial or appendicular ataxia on exam. Her gait was unstable with a notable foot drop on the left with left leg circumduction.

WHAT IS THE PACE?

This patient presents with symptom onset and evolution over the past several weeks, which fits with a subacute time course of disease.

WHAT IS THE LOCALIZATION?

First, we must decide whether her symptoms are attributable to a lesion in the central or peripheral nervous system. There are several clues in her examination that point to a central lesion, such as her up-going plantar response (or Babinski's response), but where is the lesion within the central nervous system?

We need to further characterize where in the central nervous system the lesion lies (assuming a single lesion): brain, brainstem, or spinal cord. Her examination is notable for crossed sensory and motor deficits as well as dissociated sensory tract dysfunction. Remember, the spinothalamic tracts and the dorsal columns both begin in the periphery and travel via peripheral nerves to the dorsal root ganglia (Figure 11.1). The spinothalamic tracts synapse and decussate soon after entering the spinal cord, whereas the dorsal columns synapse in the dorsal root ganglia but do not decussate until they reach the medulla. Both of these are clues to our lesion localizing to the spinal cord, especially since she has no cranial nerve abnormalities.

Of note, these findings could have easily been missed if we had not performed a more thorough sensory examination. What prompted this change in exam? As alluded to previously, this is the importance of adapting the exam to the patient's complaint and history. A patient who presents with a seizure likely does not need multiple sensory modalities tested. However, a patient who presents with weakness and numbness needs a more in-depth exam that reflects their symptoms.

We need to identify where the lesion is within the spinal cord. Can we assign one lesion in the spinal cord as the cause of all of her symptoms? It might seem daunting at first to have multiple

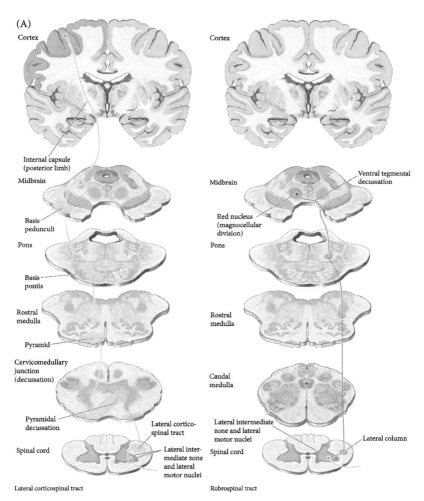

Figure 11.1. (**A**) Descending lateral corticospinal tract, (**B**) ascending spinothalamic tract, and (**C**) ascending dorsal column. Note that in the spinal cord the fibers in the spinothalamic tract are crossed and contralateral to the side of origin whereas the fibers in the dorsal column and corticospinal tracts are uncrossed and ipsilateral. *Reproduced by permission from Hal Blumenfeld, Neuroanatomy through Clinical Cases (New York, New York: Oxford University Press, 2018), 236, 277, 278.*

(B)

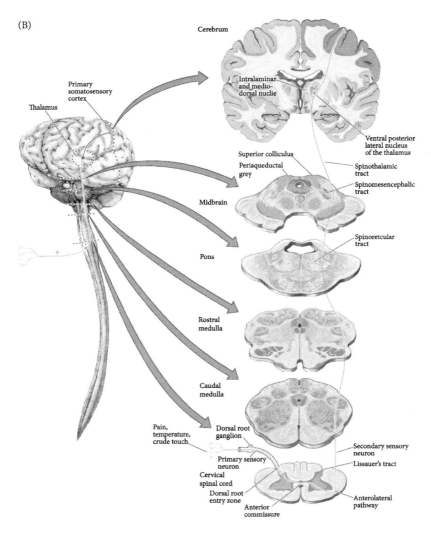

Figure 11.1. Continued

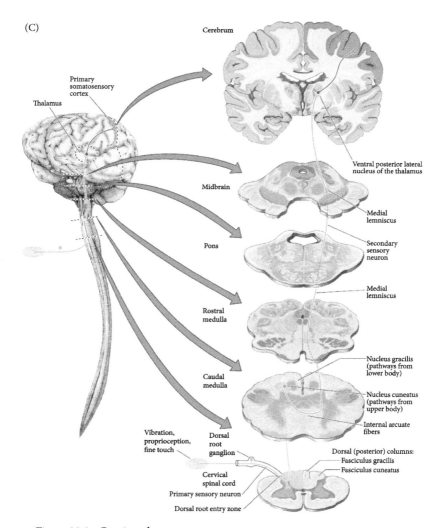

Figure 11.1. Continued

findings in her examination that are attributable to multiple different ascending and descending pathways. I advise you to start with a pathway that is familiar. Take, for example, her left leg weakness. Is a lesion in the motor fibers in the spinal cord, which make up the corticospinal tracts, ipsilateral or contralateral to the deficit? The motor signal begins in the contralateral motor cortex, but the fibers cross in the pyramidal decussation in the brainstem, leaving the corticospinal tract ipsilateral for the length of the spinal cord. Thus, we know that our lesion must involve the left side of the spinal cord. Now, we just work in reverse for the other exam findings.

Our patient also has loss of vibration in her left leg. The axons that carry sensory information of vibration and proprioception travel in the uncrossed dorsal columns, and sensory information of pain and temperature is carried in the crossed spinothalamic tracts. It's okay if you need to look up these diagrams (see Figure 11.1 and Figure 6.1), but all of the symptoms for each tract localize to the left side of the spinal cord. Our lesion involves the corticospinal, spinothalamic, and dorsal columns all on the left, so it must take up the entire left hemi-cord. The eponym for this is called Brown-Séquard syndrome.

Lastly, is the lesion in the cervical or thoracic spinal cord? Since our patient has symptoms in the upper extremities, we know that part of the cervical cord must be involved. However, her symptoms are only in the medial aspects of each forearm and fifth digits. That, plus the predominant lower extremity involvement, suggests a lower cervical cord or upper thoracic cord lesion.

That seems like a lot of work when written out, but we can save time and resources in our work-up of our patient. All we need now is to look at her cervical and thoracic spinal cord. However, before we do that, we need to generate a differential diagnosis.

WHAT IS THE SYNDROMIC DIAGNOSIS?

Our patient is a 70-year-old woman who presents with a subacute myelopathy (spinal cord injury) involving the left hemi-cord.

WHAT IS THE ETIOLOGIC DIAGNOSIS?

Given the pace of her symptoms, possible etiologic diagnoses include neoplastic, infectious, inflammatory, or metabolic disorders. Since her symptoms localize to the spinal cord, we must also consider structural disease (such as spinal stenosis or a herniated disc).

Now that we have generated our differential etiologic diagnoses, let us take a look at an MRI of her cervical and thoracic spinal cord.

ADDITIONAL INFORMATION

Her MRI (Figure 11.2) shows a lesion in her spinal cord involving the lower cervical and upper thoracic cord. If you look closely at the axial cross-section, you will see that only the left side of the cord is involved. This is exactly what we suspected based on her examination. What we don't see is any large mass or herniated disc, taking malignancy and structural spine disease off the differential. Thus, the possible etiologic diagnoses left on our differential are inflammatory or infectious disorders. However, we can't identify a specific etiology without laboratory testing.

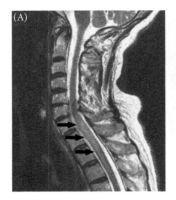
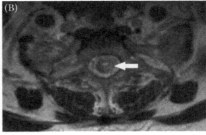

Figure 11.2. (**A**) MRI cervical spine sagittal STIR shows a longitudinally exten-sive lesion spanning her lower cervical and upper thoracic spinal cord (*arrows*). (**B**) MRI cervical spine axial T2 demonstrates a representative cross-section showing an eccentrically placed lesion in the left hemi-cord (*arrow*).

CONCLUSION

Ultimately, she was diagnosed with the pathologic diagnosis of neuromyelitis optica spectrum disorder (NMOSD) after serum testing revealed the presence of an aquaporin 4 antibody. NMOSD is an autoimmune disorder of the central nervous system. The most common sites of disease include the optic nerves and spinal cord. However, NMOSD can also cause inflammation in the area postrema, hypothalamus, and brain. Quick recognition of NMOSD is critical. The inflammatory attacks of NMOSD tend to be severe and less responsive to conventional treatment with high-dose steroids compared to multiple sclerosis. Prompt initiation of plasma exchange, which is often more effective than high-dose ste-roid monotherapy, can prevent more severe permanent neurologic disability.

Chapter 12

A man who began to drool

A 41-year-old man with a history of testicular cancer presented with headache. He initially developed several days of fatigue, a generalized tension-type headache, and the feeling that he was "hung over." Within a few days of symptom onset, he noted a burning pain over his left abdomen and right retroauricular pain. He presented for evaluation when he woke up the following day and his wife told him that his face was drooping. He noticed when he drank water from a cup it dribbled down his mouth, and he was more sensitive to sounds on the right side. He denied any fever, weight loss, or night sweats. However, he had developed a non-pruritic, erythematous rash over his chest and abdomen (Figure 12.1). He had recently traveled to Vermont for a camping trip with his family, but he otherwise denied any recent exposures.

There are several classic presentations of neurologic disease where it is absolutely critical to have a standardized exam to evaluate for a specific chief complaint. For example, in a patient who presents with foot drop, you need to test for specific features to distinguish between a neuropathy and a radiculopathy. Likewise, for a patient who presents with facial droop, you need to know which elements of the history and exam are critical to help distinguish an upper versus lower motor neuron facial droop. The differential diagnosis is vastly different and hinges on the correct localization.

Before you go any further, what are the distinguishing exam features that we should look for to distinguish an upper versus a lower motor neuron facial droop? Don't stop with just saying whether the upper face is involved. Anecdotally, I find that patients and medical professionals frequently cannot determine whether the upper face is involved or even identify the correct side of the facial weakness! There are more reliable "hard" exam findings for those who know how to look.

Figure 12.1. Representative image of the rash that was widespread over the patient's torso and back.

On examination, he had a normal mental status. He endorsed mild discomfort due to his headache. Cranial nerve examination was notable for normal visual acuity and extraocular movements.

He had normal facial sensation. He had near-complete paralysis of the right face. He could not grin on the right side. When asked to forcefully close his eyes, his right eyelid was easily opened and Bell's phenomenon was seen (discussed later). He endorsed that sounds were louder on the right side compared to the left. Corneal reflex was absent on the right but present on the left. He could not correctly identify the taste of sugar water when a droplet was placed on the right side of his tongue. The rest of his cranial nerve exam was normal. Motor exam was normal. He had burning pain and hyperpathia over the left T10 and T11 dermatomes. His reflexes were normal, and his gait was normal. His rash is shown in Figure 12.1

WHAT IS THE PACE?

He presents with symptoms that evolved over days, which is consistent with an acute to subacute onset of disease.

WHAT IS THE LOCALIZATION?

To determine an upper versus lower motor neuron facial palsy, we need to know what the facial (seventh) nerve does, and which functions it has in addition to its function as a motor nerve of the face (Figure 12.2).

First, we will start with evaluation of motor function. He has evidence of upper and lower facial weakness. I will not spend an

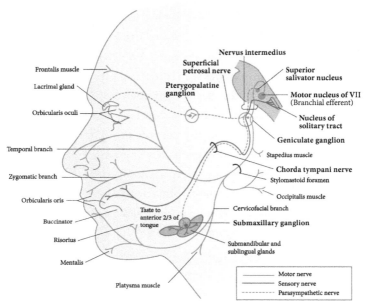

Figure 12.2. Illustration of the branches of the facial nerve and function of each branch—motor, sensory, and/or parasympathetic. *Republished with permission of McGraw Hill LLC, from* Clinical Neuroanatomy, *Stephen G. Waxman, 26th edition, 2009; permission conveyed through Copyright Clearance Center, Inc.*

inordinate amount of time discussing the anatomy behind unilateral versus bilateral innervation of the face and why an upper motor neuron lesion should spare the forehead, as that is typically covered in basic neuroanatomy. However, it is frequently surprisingly challenging for the examiner to accurately identify forehead weakness or sparing. Thus, we need alternative methods of more definitively identifying upper face weakness. He has Bell's phenomenon (palpebral oculogyric reflex) with forced eyelid closure, which is a reflex that is typically not seen unless there is facial weakness allowing the examiner to pry open the eyelid. Forced eyelid closure causes the pupils to deviate upwards. You can imagine the evolutionary advantage to this reflex: If you were trying to protect your eyes from some external threat, you would close them very tightly. The eyes deviate upwards, which further protects the pupils from potential harm. This reflex always occurs with forced eyelid closure, but it is typically only seen when the orbicularis oculi is sufficiently weak for the examiner to open the eyelid and see the pupil.

Let's move on to his other deficits. To understand these, and to know to test them, we need to think about the various afferent and efferent components of the facial nerve (see Figure 12.2). In addition to the motor function of the facial nerve to the muscles of the face, it also has a small sensory component: taste of the anterior two-thirds of the tongue. These fibers travel from the tongue along the lingual nerve, hitch a ride on the chorda tympani, and then join the facial nerve.

He has loss of the corneal reflex; mildly noxious stimuli to the right cornea does not cause him to reflexively blink. The afferent component of this reflex arc is mediated by sensory fibers in the trigeminal nerve. The efferent component of this reflex arc is mediated by motor fibers in the facial nerve.

How might we explain his changes in hearing? Why would he have increased sensitivity to sound on the right side? The facial nerve gives off the nerve to the stapedius muscle, which helps to dampen the transmission of sound by stabilizing the stapes. When the stapedius is paralyzed, such as in a seventh-nerve palsy, there is less dampening, which leads to increased volume on the side of the lesion.

In addition to these functions of the facial nerve, it also innervates various glands, such as the lacrimal gland. All of these deficits are variably present depending on where the lesion is along the facial nerve. For example, lesions of the facial nerve distal to the nerve to the stapedius will not result in hearing changes. Figure 12.2 depicts the course of the facial nerve. All of the findings we have described in our patient have objectively, and exhaustively, demonstrated that the lesion lies in the seventh cranial nerve.

The only other finding on his exam was sensory changes over his abdomen in the distribution of T10 and T11. This indicates either a radiculopathy or neuropathy involving the thoracic roots or inter-costal nerves at that level.

The presence of headache and possible dysfunction of a cra-nial nerve and thoracic roots raises the possibility that the un-derlying pathology that ties these findings together involves the spinal fluid or meninges. A leptomeningeal process could cause disease in the cranial nerves and spinal roots, which are geograph-ically separate in the neuraxis, by affecting both nerves and roots as they course through the spinal fluid after exiting the brainstem and spinal cord.

WHAT IS THE SYNDROMIC DIAGNOSIS?

He presents with acute to subacute onset of a seventh-nerve palsy and thoracic neuropathy or radiculopathy that we suspect might be due to a leptomeningeal process.

WHAT IS THE ETIOLOGIC DIAGNOSIS?

Potential etiologic diagnoses based on his pace of disease include infectious, inflammatory, and neoplastic disorders. To help us establish the underlying pathologic diagnosis of his suspected meningeal process, we will need to know some additional information.

ADDITIONAL INFORMATION

He had normal imaging of his brain and spine. His CSF showed 21 white blood cells (normal 0–5 cells/mm^3), total protein 41 (normal 18–45 mg/dL), and glucose 57 (normal 40–80 mg/dL).

CONCLUSION

There is clear evidence of inflammation in the spinal fluid. His full syndromic diagnosis is confirmed to be an acute to subacute onset of meningitis associated with facial palsy and a thoracic radiculopathy/neuropathy. Even without the *context* helping us to narrow down the possible etiologic diagnoses, we can arrive at the correct pathologic diagnosis for this disorder with a simple search on the internet (search *meningitis, facial palsy*, and *radiculopathy* if you don't believe me). However, the context here is quite helpful. He recently went on a camping trip in an area endemic with Lyme disease. In addition, his rash is consistent with multifocal erythema migrans.

Lyme disease is caused by the spirochete *Borrelia burgdorferi* in the United States. There are several other closely related species that also cause infection in Europe and Asia. The rash is caused by the hematogenous spread of spirochetes migrating radially from each nidus. Most individuals who contract Lyme disease do not have neurologic manifestations. When neurologic manifestations are present (referred to as neuroborreliosis), the typical symptoms include meningitis, cranial neuritis (most commonly unilateral or bilateral facial palsies), and radiculoneuritis. These can present independently or in various combinations. Thankfully, *Borrelia* species remain exquisitely sensitive to antibiotic therapy, and neuroborreliosis is easily treatable. He made a full recovery.

Chapter 13

A woman with pain and difficulty walking

A 65-year-old woman presented to the emergency room for evaluation of difficulty walking. She initially noted numbness and heaviness in her bilateral lower extremities 3 weeks prior to presentation. She had some mild unsteadiness while standing and walking. Over the next 3 weeks, she developed paresthesias in her bilateral toes that ascended up both legs as well as aching lower back pain. She had two episodes of fecal incontinence on the day prior to presentation. She noted loss of sensation in the perineal area. She denied any changes in sensation or strength in her bilateral upper extremities. She had no vision changes, including diplopia. She endorsed a 15-lb weight loss over the past few months. She denied any fevers, and she had not had any recent exposures or travel.

This is a concerning history. What draws your attention, and why are you concerned? Everything she reports seems like a pertinent positive, and there are multiple "red flags" for a serious illness. However, rather than using her history to jump to potential pathologic diagnoses, can these "red flags" also help us quickly localize the lesion? Try to think about why certain features of her history stand out, and what their potential localizations are. This will help us to more quickly and easily make the pathologic diagnosis.

On examination, she was well-appearing, but thin. She had a soft, several-centimeter mass over her left parietal convexity, which was non-tender. She had no surrounding skin changes or hair loss. Her mental status was normal. There were no cranial nerve abnormalities. Muscle tone was normal throughout. Her strength was normal in the upper extremities. She had hip flexor weakness (4−) bilaterally. Hip abduction and knee extension were both full strength. Knee flexion was weak, 4 on the right and 4+ on the left. Right ankle dorsiflexion strength was 4. The rest of her strength was full in the lower extremities. Sensory testing revealed diminished vibration bilaterally at the toes and impaired proprioception. She had a positive Romberg test. She had decreased tone of her anal sphincter and perineal sensory loss. Her reflexes were diminished in the bilateral lower extremities with the exception of the left Achilles reflex, which was relatively spared. Her toes were down-going. There was no dysmetria, and she walked with a wide-based gait.

WHAT IS THE PACE?

She presents with symptoms that developed over weeks, which is consistent with a subacute time course of disease.

WHAT IS THE LOCALIZATION?

She presents with gait difficulty, and her symptoms and examination reveal motor, sensory, and bowel dysfunction. Although she has weakness, she has no features of damage to the upper motor neurons—she has no spasticity, and her reflexes are diminished with down-going toes. This would seem to indicate that the lesion doesn't involve the central nervous system; rather, it localizes to the peripheral nervous system.

When a patient has multiple deficits, it is often helpful to hone in on the deficit(s) that are uncommon or have more specific localizations rather than starting with something nonspecific such as difficulty walking. In her case, her fecal incontinence, decreased anal sphincter tone, and saddle anesthesia are the most striking. All of these signs and symptoms indicate sacral dysfunction. These deficits could arise either from the lower spinal cord (such as in conus medullaris syndrome), the sacral nerve roots (such as in cauda equina syndrome), or the lumbosacral plexus. In contrast to the challenges we would run into if we attempted to start by localizing leg weakness (which could be from her cortex down to the muscle), we can immediately narrow down our localization to a few spots in nervous system (Figure 13.1).

Now, let's characterize her motor deficits. First, she has notable sparing of the upper extremities. Second, the weakness in her lower extremities involves the proximal as well as distal muscles without any apparent pattern. Third, both extremities are affected, but asymmetrically. Whenever anything is asymmetric and not length dependent, we must always think about multiple radiculopathies, a plexopathy, or multiple neuropathies. For example, if this were a myopathy, we might expect proximal muscles to be affected more than distal muscles. If this were an isolated neuropathy or radiculopathy (such as a peroneal neuropathy or L4 radiculopathy), then we might expect isolated muscle involvement or specific patterns. This asymmetric and non–length-dependent weakness in her lower

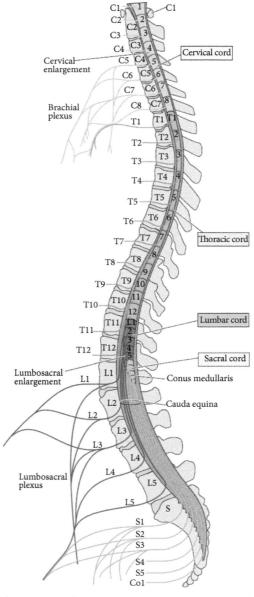

Figure 13.1. The segments of the spinal cord: cervical, thoracic, lumbar, and sacral. Note the location of the lumbosacral nerve roots in relation to the end of the spinal cord (conus medullaris). *Reproduced by permission from Hal Blumenfeld, Neuroanatomy through Clinical Cases (New York, New York: Oxford University Press, 2018), 22.*

extremities fits with either multiple lumbar radiculopathies or a lumbosacral plexopathy as discussed earlier.

We are left with a process that involves either the lumbosacral nerve roots (such as in cauda equina or conus medullaris syndrome) or a lumbosacral plexopathy. Her history includes one clue that may make a plexopathy less likely. She has aching low back pain, which is more typical of cauda equina or conus medullaris syndrome over a plexopathy. Questions that arise on examinations tend to overstate the differences in distinguishing conus medullaris and cauda equina syndrome (and even lumbosacral plexopathies). In clinical practice, there is frequently overlap of many of the symptoms of these entities, and the underlying disease may impact both the lower cord and the lumbosacral nerve roots. However, if we had to choose one final localization, perhaps a cauda equina syndrome is more likely due to three possible reasons. Can you identify any?

First, she has asymmetric motor deficits, which we might expect to be more likely in a disorder where multiple nerve roots are differentially affected rather than in the conus. Second, her reflexes are diminished as opposed to increased, which we might expect if upper motor neurons were involved. Third, her bowel dysfunction came late in the time course of disease, which is more common in cauda equina syndrome. This is not a major point and not particularly relevant in clinical practice.

WHAT IS THE DIFFERENTIAL DIAGNOSIS?

Our patient is a 65-year-old woman who presents with a syndromic diagnosis of subacute onset of a cauda equina syndrome.

WHAT IS THE ETIOLOGIC DIAGNOSIS?

The *etiologic diagnoses* for subacute neurologic syndromes in this case are relatively broad and include inflammatory, infectious, and neoplastic disorders. Undoubtedly, there is a long list of esoteric and rare disorders that could be causing this syndrome. Can the *context* of her presentation help us narrow down the differential diagnosis any further?

There are two notable features of her history and exam. The first is that she has had 15 lbs of unintentional weight loss. The second is that she has a calvarial mass. Admittedly, these can't rule in or rule out many diagnoses, but they do raise the suspicion for a neoplastic disorder, especially with the lack of context for her to have developed an infection, as the *pathologic diagnosis* of her presentation. Armed with our hypotheses, we can now obtain appropriate imaging to evaluate for a potentially neoplastic disease causing a cauda equina syndrome.

CONCLUSION

Unfortunately, her imaging (Figure 13.2) confirmed our hypothesis of the pathologic diagnosis.

We can see extensive, bulky leptomeningeal disease along the surface of the conus medullaris and the cauda equina. There is diffuse contrast enhancement. The arrows show several examples of the bulky nodularity of the nerve roots, which is quite striking. In addition, there are diffuse bone marrow signal abnormalities as well as an L2 pathologic fracture. All of these findings are highly

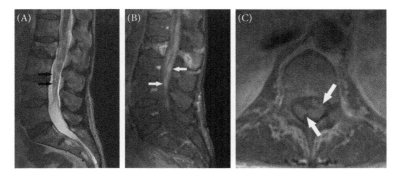

Figure 13.2. (**A**) MRI lumbar spine sagittal T2, (**B**) MRI lumbar spine sagittal T1 post-contrast, and (**C**) MRI lumbar spine T1 post-contrast. The *arrows* point to several examples of the severe, nodular contrast-enhancing lumbosacral nerve roots.

concerning for a malignant neoplasm. She was ultimately diagnosed with B-cell non-Hodgkin's lymphoma with widespread bone, bone marrow, and leptomeningeal lymphomatosis.

Chapter 14

A woman who collapsed
in a train station

A 45-year-old woman with a history of epilepsy and cerebral palsy was brought to the hospital by EMS after bystanders witnessed her suddenly collapse and start shaking in all of her extremities. She had a history of intractable epilepsy with breakthrough seizures on levetiracetam. She had recently been seen in clinic by her neurologist, who had switched her to valproate from levetiracetam.

When she was initially seen in the emergency room, she was lying face down in bed. It took much encouragement to get her to turn over. She could follow simple commands. She was intermittently screaming and crying. Her speech was thick with dysarthria.

Her initial evaluation in the emergency room was notable for an undetectable level of valproate in her blood. Toxicology screen was negative. She had a 30-minute EEG, which showed bi-frontal sharp discharges but no active seizures (consistent with her known history of epilepsy). She had a head CT, which was unremarkable. The emergency room staff then witnessed a

45-second generalized convulsion. She was given lorazepam and levetiracetam.

We are going to do this case slightly differently. We will go through the routine of identifying the pace and localization, but we will do it stepwise as the case unfolds.

WHAT IS THE PACE?

She presents with multiple episodes of sudden-onset change in mental status with convulsive activity that has an onset of mere seconds. This is consistent with a hyperacute pace.

WHAT IS THE LOCALIZATION?

As discussed in Chapter 7, we can localize consciousness to certain regions of the nervous system. Remember, the ascending reticular arousal system (RAS) comprises the upper brainstem, thalamus, hypothalamus, basal forebrain, and cortex. For a lesion to cause coma (such as in this case), the lesion must be large enough in any of these areas to cause sufficient disruption to the RAS. In this case, we don't have any features on history or examination that can clearly point us to one part of the nervous system, but, in the absence of any focal deficits, we must rely on the *context* to help us localize the lesion. In this case, the context of her history of epilepsy and recent changes in medication points to a localization of bilateral cortical dysfunction due to a generalized tonic-clonic seizure.

WHAT IS THE DIFFERENTIAL DIAGNOSIS?

The algorithmic approach to acute medical emergencies necessitates we rule out "can't miss" diagnoses (such as intracranial hemorrhage, drug overdose, status epilepticus), but her initial evaluation did not reveal any conditions that could have been responsible for her presentation. Since the algorithmic approach to evaluation did not reveal a known etiology, let's go back to pace and localization.

She presents with hyperacute onset of a process that causes coma (disruption of the RAS). As mentioned, without the context it is hard to definitively localize and identify the syndromic diagnosis. However, given the context of a woman with known epilepsy with witnessed convulsions who may not be on any anti-epileptic medications based on blood testing, the top of our differential of etiologic diagnoses must be seizure.

We are ready to move on to the next part of her hospital course.

An individual who presents with multiple generalized convulsions may have a prolonged post-ictal phase lasting for hours. Based on her initial evaluation, she was admitted to the hospital for further management and observation of a suspected post-ictal state.

Overnight, and several hours after her last witnessed convulsion in the emergency room, she had a repeat neurologic exam. This time, her eyes were closed and did not open to noxious stimuli. Her pupils were 1.5 mm bilaterally with trace reactivity. She had a right exotropia, and a central gaze with absent vestibulo-ocular reflex (VOR). She could localize to noxious

stimuli in her upper extremities, and she could withdraw to noxious stimuli in her lower extremities. Babinski's sign was present
bilaterally.

Does this additional neurologic exam help us to better localize
her lesion? Remember that earlier in the case we did not have a
clear localization to her decreased arousal. Based on the context, we
assumed (not unreasonably so) that the etiology of her presentation
was due to seizure. Take a minute to think about the exam prior to
reading the rest of the case. Can you identify a lesion in the nervous
system that could explain these findings as well as her decreased
arousal?

The next morning, now approximately 16 hours after her initial presentation, she was unresponsive to noxious stimuli. Her
heart rate oscillated between bradycardia (as low as 30 beats per
minute) to tachycardia (as high as 120 beats per minute). Her
pupils were pinpoint and non-reactive. Her extremities were in
tonic extensor posturing.

WHAT IS THE LOCALIZATION?

Now that we have additional information, let's try to more fully localize the lesion.

A commonly used expression is that the eye is a window to the
brain. Detecting abnormalities in pupil size, position, or movement
is sometimes all that is needed to localize a lesion. She has fixed,
pinpoint pupils. Pupillary constriction and dilation are regulated
by the parasympathetic and sympathetic fibers. Parasympathetic
fibers from the midbrain carried by the oculomotor nerves cause

pupillary constriction. Sympathetic fibers that dilate the pupil take a more circuitous route. First-order neurons descend through the brainstem to the thoracic spine. There, they synapse and second-order neurons ascend through the thoracic ganglion to the superior cervical ganglion. Third-order (post-ganglionic) neurons then travel up the carotid plexus to the pupil. She has constricted and non-reactive pupils; thus, we know that she has interruption of the sympathetic fibers somewhere along this pathway.

Let's now turn our focus to her absent VOR, commonly referred to as having "doll's eyes." First, we need to know what this means. When trying to understand various reflexes, I find it is helpful to first think about the evolutionary necessity of the reflex. The VOR refers to the involuntary conjugate eye movements that occur equal and opposite to turning one's head. Why is this a critical function? We need to be able to maintain fixation on a target despite normal vertical and horizontal head turning that constantly occurs. Imagine trying to walk if you couldn't keep your eyes focused on a target and your vision bounced up and down with every small movement of your head. Alternatively, imagine trying to hunt an animal while running if you constantly had visual slip from slight movements of your head if you ran. We would not get very far in the world without the ability to maintain fixation thanks to the VOR.

When we test the VOR with a horizontal head turn, what are we testing? Figure 14.1 depicts the horizontal VOR. First, we need to know that the head is turning in the horizontal plane (the afferent limb to the reflex arc). That is the role of the vestibular system, so cranial nerve VIII is involved. Next, the eyes need to turn equal and opposite to the rotation of the head (the efferent limb of the reflex arc). That means one eye must abduct and the other eye adducts (which eye depends on the direction of the head turn). To accomplish this, cranial nerves III and VI are involved. Since this is *absent*

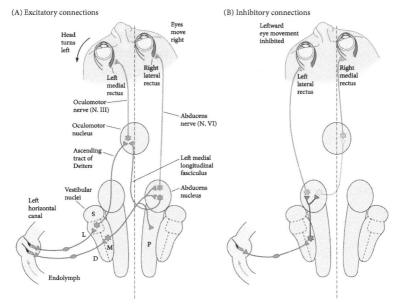

Figure 14.1. Illustration of the neuroanatomy of the horizontal vestibulo-ocular reflex (VOR). A head turn causes endolymph to flow in the horizontal canal. This signal is carried via the vestibular nerve to the brainstem to activate the ipsilateral medial rectus (via the oculomotor nerve) and the contralateral lateral rectus (via the abducens nerve). An equal inhibitory signal is sent to the contralateral muscle pairs. *Republished with permission of McGraw Hill LLC, from* Principles of Neural Science, *Kandel, Eric R., James H. Schwartz, Thomas M. Jessell, Steven A. Siegelbaum, and A.J. Hudspeth, 5th edition, 2012; permission conveyed through Copyright Clearance Center, Inc.*

on her examination, we know that some part of this reflex arc is impaired (either the afferent or efferent limb or both).

We now have enough evidence to definitively localize the lesion. She has coma, pinpoint pupils, and an impaired VOR. The lesion must be in the brainstem. Specifically, we are worried about the pons. This could cause impaired arousal to the reticular arousing system, pinpoint pupils, and impaired horizontal VOR. There are other features that are also consistent with a brainstem lesion, such as her posturing, autonomic instability, and positive Babinski's sign. However, we will not go into those in depth in this case.

WHAT IS THE SYNDROMIC DIAGNOSIS?

Unfortunately, our syndromic diagnosis is now very different than what we first thought. She presents with hyperacute onset of a brainstem (pontine) lesion.

WHAT IS THE ETIOLOGIC DIAGNOSIS?

Since seizures localize to the cortex and her symptoms localize to the brainstem, that can no longer be the etiology of her presentation. The only etiologic diagnosis that fits with the hyperacute onset of a brainstem syndrome is vascular (either ischemic or hemorrhagic stroke). However, we know that there is no hemorrhage, as that would have been seen on her initial head CT.

CONCLUSION

Unfortunately, MRI diffusion-weighted imaging (Figure 14.2) showed what we suspected.

She had suffered an acute ischemic stroke in her upper pons. This case is a devastating example of cognitive bias in medicine. We see the risk of anchoring and the framing effect of the initial context of her presentation. Her history provided the perfect context for a breakthrough seizure. She had a known history of epilepsy. She had

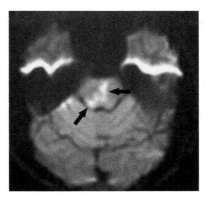

Figure 14.2. MRI brain axial DWI at the level of the pons. The *arrows* point to an area of restricted diffusion consistent with acute infarction.

recently changed her anti-epileptic treatment. Her levels of her anti-epileptic treatments were undetectable. She had witnessed events that were reported as seizures.

One of the most important roles of establishing the *pace* and *localization* is that it helps us to avoid cognitive biases that could potentially lead us astray. In this case, even though a very appropriate neurologic exam was performed overnight, cognitive biases may have delayed the final diagnosis.

Lastly, you might be wondering what the convulsive episodes were that so many individuals witnessed. Brainstem, in particular pontine, infarcts can cause convulsive movements, both focal and generalized, that can mimic epileptic seizures.

Chapter 15

A man with symptoms that improved throughout the day

A 74-year-old man presented for evaluation due to recent onset of difficulty walking. He describes that his initial symptom was episodic vertigo, which began 1 month prior. He was diagnosed with benign positional paroxysmal vertigo (BPPV), for which he was treated, but his vertigo worsened. Approximately 1 week after onset of vertigo, he developed nausea and difficulty walking. He began having retro-orbital headaches that would wake him from sleep. On the week prior to presentation, he had episodes of emesis and hiccups, and he was unable to walk due to feeling unstable on his feet. His wife reported that he appeared excessively sleepy and that his thinking was not clear. Over the course of the month, all of his symptoms progressively became more intense, and they all tended to be worse in the morning after awakening and improve later in the day.

He was initially diagnosed with BPPV after presenting with vertigo, but he quickly develops additional symptoms that draw that diagnosis into question. What features of the history help you distinguish between a "central" versus a "peripheral" cause of his vertigo? In addition, what warning signs are present in the history that point to a potentially life-threatening process? Sometimes the history helps to localize the lesion based on not just the symptoms the patient reports, but also the manner or circumstances in which the symptoms present. How does the fact that his symptoms are worse in the morning and improve throughout the day help us localize the lesion?

On examination, he was awake, alert, and oriented. He had mildly restricted up-gaze bilaterally. There were no other abnormalities with extraocular movements. He had mild swelling of his optic discs bilaterally. All other cranial nerves were normal. His strength was full throughout, and his sensation was normal. He had dysmetria with finger-to-nose and heel-to-shin bilaterally, but worse on the right side compared to the left side. Reflexes were normal. He had a wide-based, ataxic gait, and he was unable to tandem walk.

WHAT IS THE PACE?

He initially developed vertigo 1 month prior to admission, and then he had new and progressively worsening symptoms over the following 4 weeks. This fits with a subacute pace of disease.

WHAT IS THE LOCALIZATION?

We do not need to belabor the localization of his gait ataxia and dysmetria in this case, since we covered it in Chapter 8. These symptoms are most likely due to a lesion in the cerebellum. His vertigo may also localize to the cerebellum, although there were no features on exam to help distinguish between a cerebellar and a vestibular origin of his vertigo. His nausea and emesis could also be due to a cerebellar lesion or to elevated intracranial pressure (ICP), as discussed later in this chapter.

The localization and the function of hiccups are not fully understood. However, when due to a primary CNS pathology, hiccups develop secondary to lesions of the medulla or posterior fossa or due to elevated intracranial pressure. What we do not see on his exam is any evidence of a medullary syndrome, making intrinsic brainstem pathology less likely. However, he has limited up-gaze on his exam, and his headaches are exacerbated by lying down (such as at night when he is asleep). These warning signs, in addition to swelling of his optic discs on his exam, tell us that his headaches and hiccups are likely due to elevated ICP. Of note, papilledema refers to swelling of the optic disc secondary to elevated ICP. There are other disorders that cause swelling of the optic discs (such as inflammation of the optic nerve head). Unless elevated ICP is suspected or confirmed to be the cause of optic nerve head swelling, then we should not use the term papilledema.

Let's summarize the localization. He has evidence of cerebellar dysfunction as well as signs and symptoms of elevated ICP. Thus, we might expect him to have a space-occupying lesion in the cerebellum exerting mass effect and leading to elevated ICP.

WHAT IS THE SYNDROMIC DIAGNOSIS?

He presents with subacute onset of symptoms most characteristic of a cerebellar lesion with mass effect leading to elevated ICP.

WHAT IS THE ETIOLOGIC DIAGNOSIS?

The etiologic differential based on our syndromic diagnosis includes infectious, inflammatory, and neoplastic conditions. Other causes, such as metabolic or toxic etiologies, are less likely due to the features of the history and exam that raise concern for a space-occupying lesion in the posterior fossa. For example, it would be unlikely for alcoholic cerebellar degeneration to cause cerebellar edema leading to elevated ICP. Since we expect a space-occupying lesion, then we expect imaging to be abnormal and, hopefully, guide us to the correct diagnosis.

ADDITIONAL INFORMATION

An MRI of his brain (Figure 15.1) showed edema in the right cerebellar hemisphere that resulted in partial effacement of the fourth

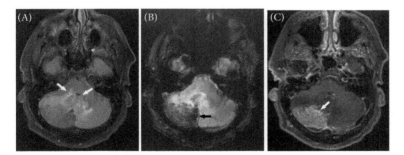

Figure 15.1. (**A**) MRI brain axial FLAIR, (**B**) axial GRE, and (**C**) axial T1 post-contrast images. There is edema with mass effect and midline shift (*arrows*). The lesion is hypointense on GRE, indicating hemorrhage, and there is contrast enhancement.

ventricle. In addition, there was hemosiderin deposition within the lesion, which indicated prior hemorrhage.

A CT angiogram (not pictured here) showed an absence of the right posterior inferior cerebellar artery. Based on the findings seen on MRI and CT, the neuroradiologists believed the most likely diagnosis was a subacute infarct in the distribution of the right posterior inferior cerebellar artery with hemorrhagic conversion.

WHAT IS THE DIFFERENTIAL DIAGNOSIS?

Did this patient have an ischemic stroke with hemorrhagic conversion as suspected by his imaging? Let's go back to pace and localization. An ischemic stroke *should* be hyperacute. We might be able to accept some ambiguity in the history and allow for a slightly longer timeframe, but a history of progressive symptoms over the course of the month just doesn't fit with an ischemic stroke. We could try to make the argument that the ischemic stroke had a hyperacute onset and that his symptoms worsened due to hemorrhage and edema that subsequently developed within the stroke bed. This isn't unreasonable—but still, a time course of 1 month just seems far too long. There is a clinical and radiographic disconnect. The principles of pace and localization tell us that the lesion we see on MRI is unlikely to be a stroke. Our etiologic diagnosis should be an infectious, inflammatory, or neoplastic process.

Due to his progressively worsening symptoms, concern for increased edema, and the potential for the development of hydrocephalus and herniation, he went to the operating room for a biopsy and decompressive craniotomy. The final pathology results were consistent with hemorrhage and ischemic changes. There was no tumor or significant inflammatory infiltrate. Is this an exception to the rules we established at the beginning of the book? Was his entire presentation really due to a stroke?

CLINICAL COURSE AND ADDITIONAL INFORMATION

He was seen in clinic approximately 1 month later. He endorsed persistent ataxia, vertigo, and nausea, but his symptoms concerning for elevated ICP (such as headaches that awoke him from sleep and hiccups) had fully resolved. A repeat MRI of his brain showed persistent edema, hemorrhage, and contrast enhancement. Now the neuroradiologists did not think a stroke was the likely cause, since there was no improvement on his MRI compared to a month prior. We would expect a stroke to change and resolve over time. What could this be? It isn't a stroke because the pace of symptoms never fit, and the persistently abnormal MRI doesn't fit. The biopsy didn't show a tumor or other definitive pathologic diagnosis.

CONCLUSION

In the end, this case did "break the rules." His symptoms were not due to a tumor, an infection, or any other disease that you would find listed in the etiologies of disease found in Table 1.1 in the first chapter. The cerebral angiogram (Figure 15.2) depicts arterial-to-venous shunting and an early cerebral vein. These subtle findings, not detected on any prior imaging, revealed the final diagnosis: a cerebellar pial arteriovenous fistula or arteriovenous malformation.

Ultimately, his presentation was due to a vascular phenomenon, albeit not a classic arterial ischemic or hemorrhagic stroke.

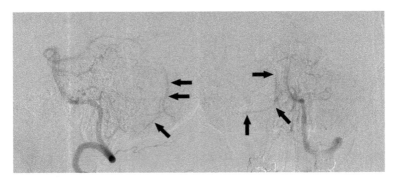

Figure 15.2. Representative images from his conventional angiogram obtained on follow-up approximately 1 month after his initial presentation. The *arrows* depict subtle arterial-to-venous shunting and an early cerebral vein.

As mentioned in the introduction, venous thromboses, AVMs, and arteriovenous fistulas can present with any pace of onset, from hyperacute to chronic. The pace can be prolonged when the symptoms are due to edema or venous (low-pressure) congestion or hemorrhage. The pace is typically hyperacute or acute when there is arterial hemorrhage. These can be notoriously difficult to diagnosis, as they may not be readily apparent on CT or MRI.

Not every case fits nicely into the framework of pace and localization. The take-home message from this case is that atypical syndromic diagnoses that "break the rules" should be considered when there is a discrepancy between the history and exam with the ancillary data that have been collected.

Chapter 16

A woman who bit her nails in public

A 64-year-old right-handed woman had an episode where she was unable to recognize one of her long-time coworkers. Over the next several years, her daughter observed the patient to have delayed verbal and motor responses and a flat affect. She stopped driving independently because she would frequently become disoriented even in familiar environments around her home. Three years after her first symptoms, she became progressively more disinhibited. She frequently bit her nails in public and would spit them on the floor. Her family could no longer take her to restaurants because she would insist on walking in circles around the dining room. She also became physically aggressive with her husband. Her daughter observed her continuing to talk on the phone even after the call had ended. She could no longer understand complex sentences when speaking with her family. The patient had no insight into these symptoms. She remained independent of all activities of daily living, managed her own finances, and worked several days per week as a hair stylist for 4 years after her initial symptoms. She also remained physically active, exercising multiple times per week, until she suffered a right humeral fracture due to a fall.

A rich history, although incredibly helpful in forming a diagnosis and guiding the subsequent physical examination, can be daunting. In some cases, such as this one, the history squarely points to multiple symptoms related to cognitive dysfunction. The key is to focus on not only what specific cognitive domains are abnormal but also what specific cognitive domains are normal, or at least much more so. This can be a helpful clue as to the localization (and etiology) of the disease. The purpose of the exam is often to corroborate and translate the symptoms the patient experiences with specific cognitive domains. Lastly, just as with other cases, which may not have as detailed of a history, the order of onset of symptoms is critical.

Take a moment to think about what you might test on your exam. A detailed cognitive examination can be tricky, and it is not intuitive. When reading the following examination, think about why certain functions were tested based on the history just given. Picture the mental status examination as a pyramid. The base levels comprise arousal, orientation, attention, and language. On top of those base levels sits memory, both short-term and long-term. Complex cognitive tasks, such as calculation, construction, and abstraction, sit at the top. Without an intact base, it is often fruitless to test the top functions. The converse also holds true: If a patient can fluently provide you a detailed history and is still working in a cognitively challenging job, there is likely no need for you to test arousal or orientation.

On examination, she was awake, alert, and oriented. She was attentive, and she had only minimal impairment of language function. Verbal memory testing was good, and short-term recall was only mildly impaired. She was unable to copy a complex figure or judge the orientation of objects. Her up-gaze was restricted. She had decreased dexterity of the left hand with increased tone and a resting tremor. Her left hand frequently fidgeted and grasped at objects next to her, which frustrated her and appeared out of her volitional control. She had palmomental reflexes bilaterally and a persistent glabellar reflex. Her gait was slow and cautious.

A CT scan of her head was unremarkable.

WHAT IS THE PACE?

Her symptoms evolved over years, so the pace is chronic.

WHAT IS THE LOCALIZATION?

We know based on the history and exam that the localization must be to the central nervous system, specifically the brain. However, in this case, identifying the specific features of cognitive dysfunction, and their individual localizations, will help guide us to the diagnosis. In broadest terms, our patient presents with dementia, which is an umbrella term for a progressive impairment in cognition such as memory, personality, and other intellectual abilities. The key to eventually generating an *etiologic diagnosis* is to identify the precise dementia syndrome.

Let's work our way first through the history and then through the exam and try to identify the individual cognitive domains that are most affected and those that are unaffected. We will then attempt to localize these to specific parts of the cerebrum. The end goal will be to generate a pattern of cerebral dysfunction that will order our differential diagnosis. Before reading further, if you haven't already done so, go back to the vignette and try to identify the key clinical features within her symptoms and exam as well as some functions that might be unaffected.

Prior to identifying the facets of cognition that are affected, let's focus on what is unaffected. As mentioned, her memory is almost completely unaffected. This striking "pertinent negative" is highly unexpected if this were to be a more typical syndrome of progressive cognitive dysfunction. This immediately indicates that the primary localization to her syndrome is *not* in the hippocampi.

One of the most striking features of her history is a change in personality and lack of self-control. The frontal lobes' proposed primary purpose is to control goal-directed behavior (previously discussed in Chapter 10). Dysfunction in the frontal lobes may manifest in varied lack of goal-directed behavior, whether it be loss of saccadic eye movements due to disruption of the frontal eye fields or an inability to maintain appropriate relationships or social behavior. Lesions in the frontal lobe can present with symptoms similar to those of our patient, who suffers from loss of inhibitory self-control and obligate reflexes (palmomental, glabellar). She also has difficulty with complex tasks, which again might represent a diminished ability to sustain goal-directed mental tasks.

Let's now pivot to some of the motor dysfunction found on examination. The most striking feature of her exam is that her left hand appears to act out of her volitional control in addition to having decreased dexterity. This is commonly referred to as "alien hand syndrome," and it can be due to various lesions involving the posterior parietal cortex. In addition, she has increased tone on the left and a resting tremor, both of which might be signs of extrapyramidal involvement and indicate dysfunction in the basal ganglia (see Chapter 9 for further discussion).

Her repeated spatial disorientation, while potentially attributable to many disorders of cognition, could be considered *topographagnosia*, or the inability to orient herself within familiar surroundings. That and her inability to recreate a complex figure, a form of *constructional apraxia*, both localize to the nondominant parietal lobe. Lesions in the nondominant parietal lobe may also cause visual disorientation.

Let's put all of this together.

WHAT IS THE SYNDROMIC DIAGNOSIS?

The syndromic diagnosis is a chronically progressive illness that localizes to the frontal lobe(s), nondominant parietal lobe, and basal ganglia. Another way to frame her localization is that she has chronically progressive asymmetric cortical and extrapyramidal dysfunction.

WHAT IS THE ETIOLOGIC DIAGNOSIS?

In the context of her age and the slow but inexorable pace of her illness, the most likely etiology is a neurodegenerative disorder. Other etiologies, such as a slow-growing benign brain tumor, are possible, but she had a negative CT that ruled out a space-occupying lesion. Thus, our etiologic diagnosis must be a neurodegenerative process that can somehow cause widespread but *asymmetric* dysfunction of wide parts of the cerebrum and basal ganglia. Now all we need to do is check to see if there is a neurodegenerative illness that matches that description. Is there?

CONCLUSION

An FDG-PET (Figure 16.1) showed striking hypometabolism throughout the right frontal and parietal lobes, which we predicted based on her history and exam.

Corticobasal syndrome is the clinical syndrome of asymmetric cortical and basal ganglionic dysfunction. The hallmark disease that causes corticobasal syndrome is corticobasal degeneration, a neuro-degenerative *tauopathy* (similar to other neurodegenerative diseases such as frontotemporal dementia or progressive supranuclear palsy). However, what sets it apart from these other tauopathies is the typical clinical syndrome of strikingly asymmetric cortical and basal ganglionic dysfunction. Corticobasal syndrome (the syndromic

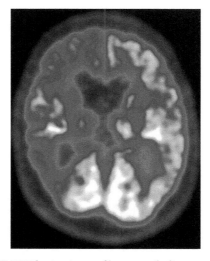

Figure 16.1. FDG-PET brain. Areas of hypometabolism appear as a dark blue or purple. Most of the cortex of the right hemisphere, excluding the occipital lobe, shows marked hypometabolism when compared to the cortex of the left hemisphere.

diagnosis) is sometimes due to other *pathologic diagnoses* such as Alzheimer's disease. The semantic distinction between corticobasal syndrome and corticobasal degeneration mirrors the pathologic distinction. Ultimately, this patient was diagnosed with corticobasal degeneration.

Chapter 17

A woman who fell in the shower

A 43-year-old woman with no significant past medical history fell in the shower. She went to the emergency room, where she was diagnosed with a mid-foot sprain and was discharged home. While attempting to recover from her injury she noted that her legs and hands felt "stiff." Over the next month, her ability to walk deteriorated to the point at which she could no longer get up the stairs on her own. Within 2 months, she was using a wheelchair. She had pain and numbness in her hands and feet that would wake her up at night. She also described a sensation of being unable to feel where her fingers and toes were in space. She stopped being able to write, type, or pick objects out of her purse.

Gait dysfunction can be due to numerous neurologic abnormalities spanning the entirety of the neuraxis. It is critical to use the history to try to define what is driving this very common symptom. What neurologic systems are involved in gait (extrapyramidal, cerebellar, motor, sensory, visual, etc.), and are there symptoms that localize to those particular systems? Breaking down the end symptom into root causes can help target your exam in this type of situation. This is not always possible based on the history, and sometimes there are no shortcuts but to do a thorough examination.

Her examination was notable for a papular rash over her hands and around her mouth. Her mental status and cranial nerves were normal. She had normal strength and muscle tone in all extremities. She had absent reflexes throughout. She had complete loss of all sensory modalities in all extremities and her chest, abdomen, and back. With her eyes closed, she had total loss of proprioception not just in her fingers and toes, but also up to her hips and shoulders. When she closed her eyes, she developed a dance-like writhing movement of her extremities. This was not present with her eyes open. She had a positive Romberg test.

WHAT IS THE PACE?

Her symptoms evolved over weeks to months, which is consistent with a subacute onset of disease.

WHAT IS THE LOCALIZATION?

This case is all about the localization. First, we need to define if the process is peripheral or central. The key features of her examination are a profound loss of sensation and reflexes with preservation of motor function. Her sensory deficits involve all extremities as well as her chest, abdomen, and back. Such a severe loss of sensation as well as areflexia points toward a problem in the peripheral nervous system. A lesion in the central nervous system would require widespread damage to bilateral hemispheres, the brainstem, or spinal cord while somehow not causing any other neurologic dysfunction. In addition, her absent reflexes are indicative of a lesion in the peripheral nervous system. Now we need to determine where the lesion is in the peripheral nervous system, which can be divided into the lower motor neurons, spinal nerves, dorsal root ganglia, brachial and lumbosacral plexi, peripheral nerves, neuromuscular junction, and muscles.

The most striking feature of her exam is the degree of sensory dysfunction with preservation of motor function. Since she has no motor deficits, the lesion cannot involve the muscles, neuromuscular junction, or lower motor neurons, since lesions in all of those places would cause weakness or other motor symptoms. Can the lesion involve the peripheral nerves? It might not be immediately obvious, but the answer is essentially no. Remember, although there are nerves that are purely sensory and others that are purely motor, the vast majority of peripheral nerves in the body carry both sensory and motor information. To have a process with such widespread sensory symptoms due to peripheral nerve disease, we would expect to see some component of motor dysfunction. This same principle means that her lesion cannot involve the brachial or lumbosacral plexus, which carry both motor and sensory fibers. Determining the localization of her lesion relies on our ability to identify where in the peripheral nervous system sensory information is located independent from motor information.

There are several different types of sensory receptors in the skin and muscles, which transmit information about pain, temperature, touch, and proprioception. These receptors transmit information up sensory axons, which travel together to make up part of the peripheral nerves and the brachial and lumbosacral plexus. The most proximal aspects of the peripheral nervous system prior to the division of sensory and motor information are the ventral and dorsal rami and spinal nerves (Figure 17.1).

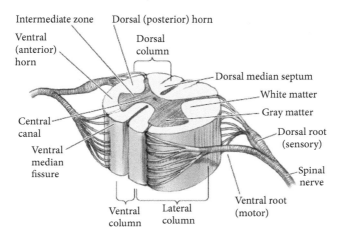

Figure 17.1. An illustrative cross-section of the spinal cord depicting the ventral and dorsal nerve roots and sensory dorsal root ganglia. *Reproduced by permission from Hal Blumenfeld, Neuroanatomy through Clinical Cases (New York, New York: Oxford University Press, 2018), 22.*

If you remember from neuroanatomy, the spinal nerves are made of a ventral root and a dorsal root, which carry motor and sensory information, respectively. The dorsal root ganglia, bipolar neurons whose axons extend into the periphery and spinal cord, are located here. These bipolar neurons within the dorsal root ganglia only carry sensory information. Thus, the only place our lesion can be in the peripheral nervous system, where sensory information is independent from motor information, is in the dorsal root ganglia.

You might have at first read her exam and thought about diseases such as Guillain–Barré syndrome, which is an autoimmune acute to subacute demyelinating polyradiculoneuropathy. This is a good first thought as it can present with similar symptoms; however, it cannot be the diagnosis in this case, since a polyradiculoneuropathy should have motor involvement.

In real life, it can sometimes be challenging to distinguish the localization of these two disorders, as severe loss of proprioception can give the false impression of weakness due to the challenges of confrontational strength testing when the patient has loss of sensation. Thus, although the localization might be highly suspected based on history and examination, diagnosing these conditions usually requires electrodiagnostic testing (Table 17.1). In our patient, sensory nerve action potentials (SNAPs) were absent in the bilateral upper and lower extremities. Motor responses and EMG (not shown) were completely normal. Isolated sensory involvement without motor nerve or muscle involvement confirmed the localization of a dorsal root ganglionopathy.

WHAT IS THE SYNDROMIC DIAGNOSIS?

Let's put the pace and localization together. The syndromic diagnosis is a subacute illness with symptoms that localize to the dorsal root ganglia.

WHAT IS THE ETIOLOGIC DIAGNOSIS?

Just like the roots and peripheral nerves in Guillain–Barré syndrome are subject to autoimmune disorders, so are the dorsal root ganglia. Given our subacute time course, our diagnosis is most likely either an autoimmune, infectious, metabolic, or toxic dorsal root ganglionopathy. A paraneoplastic syndrome is also possible, but direct neoplastic invasion would be highly unlikely to have a cancer invading only the dorsal root ganglia, and not be involving any other

Table 17.1 SENSORY NERVE CONDUCTION STUDY

Nerve/Sites	Distance (cm)	Peak latency (ms)	Amplitude (μV)
Right radial—snuff box			
Forearm	10	No response	No response
Left radial—snuff box			
Forearm	10	4.0	4.7
Left antebrachial cutaneous nerve of the forearm—lateral			
Elbow	10	No response	No response
Right sural—lateral malleolus			
Calf	14	No response	No response
Left sural—lateral malleolus			
Calf	14	No response	No response
Right superficial peroneal			
Lateral leg	14	No response	No response
Left superficial peroneal			
Lateral leg	14	No response	No response

aspect of the nervous system. Thankfully, by the time we get to our syndromic diagnosis of a dorsal root ganglionopathy, although we are left with a host of uncommon maladies (such as pyridoxine intoxication, cis-platinum toxicity, and herpes zoster, among others) the list of potential pathologic diagnoses is relatively short.

CONCLUSION

Ultimately, she was diagnosed with an autoimmune dorsal root ganglionopathy, which is commonly associated with Sjögren's syndrome. Her work-up for the rash included a skin biopsy, which was consistent with connective tissue disease, and a lip biopsy that diagnosed Sjögren's syndrome. She was treated with immunotherapy, and she had a marked improvement in her neurologic function. She regained the ability to walk, and her sensation returned, although she was left with some residual neuropathic pain. Unfortunately, many patients with a dorsal root ganglionopathy have refractory symptoms with little improvement.

Chapter 18

A woman with cough and neurologic deterioration

A 66-year-old right-handed woman with a past history of allo-genic hematopoietic stem cell transplantation for myelodysplastic syndrome presented with headache and vision changes. She was initially admitted to the hospital with fever, fatigue, and a new cough for which she received antibiotics for bacterial pneumonia. While admitted to the hospital, she had sudden onset of a right-sided headache, vision changes, and confusion. Her condition deteriorated over the next several days. She developed plegia of her left arm and leg followed by the left lower face. Unfortunately, she eventually became unarousable to stimuli.

Patients with very striking medical histories are at risk for both common and rare neurologic diseases. Since the context sets the stage for a wide differential diagnosis, defining the neurologic syndrome is critical. Don't be too engrossed with her past medical history for now. Let's stick to the basics. What do you think about the pace? Is there anything peculiar?

On her initial neurologic exam after the sudden onset of headache and vision changes, she was found to be alert and oriented to date but not location. She was inattentive, and she could only follow simple commands. Her speech was fluent. She had a right gaze preference and a left homonymous hemianopia. Other cranial nerves were unremarkable. She had a mild left hemiparesis (arm weaker than leg). She had preserved sensation but extinction on the left to double simultaneous sensory stimulation. When asked to clap, she would bring her right hand to midline and "clap" the air; her left hand remained still on the bed. Her sensation and reflexes were normal. Her subsequent examinations over the next several days were notable for decreased arousal as well as development of left lower facial droop and complete plegia of her left arm and leg.

WHAT IS THE PACE?

This one is a bit tricky. How would you define the pace? The onset of her symptoms is "sudden," so that fits with a hyperacute pace of disease. However, she subsequently worsens over the next several days. Should we still consider the pace to be hyperacute, or does this mean that the pace is acute? Could it be both? There are always exception to the rules. For now, let's consider the pace to be hyperacute, but don't forget that she progressively worsened over the next few days.

WHAT IS THE LOCALIZATION?

There is no ambiguity that this is a central rather than peripheral nervous system process. She has a right-sided headache, which indicates that the lesion is likely on the right side. In addition, she has a left homonymous hemianopia, indicating dysfunction along the visual pathway somewhere behind the optic chiasm. Be careful not to immediately assume this is dysfunction of the contralateral occipital lobe, as a more anterior thalamic lesion or a large hemispheric lesion could also cause a homonymous hemianopia.

In addition to her visual field deficit, she has signs of left-sided neglect. She has extinction to double simultaneous stimulation and Eastchester clapping sign. When asked to clap, individuals with neglect due to a right parietal lesion will bring their right hand to midline in the air in a clapping motion, but their left hand will remain limp at their side. In contrast, when patients with left upper extremity weakness due to corticospinal tract dysfunction are asked to clap, they will bring their right hand all the way over to the weak left hand to clap the two hands together. She also is disoriented to location but not time, which is atypical (usually patients are disoriented to time before location). This finding also indicates a nondominant parietal lesion.

Both her left homonymous hemianopia and left-sided neglect strongly point to a lesion involving the right parietal +/− occipital lobes. Her left hemiparesis as well as gaze preference, although potentially localizable to other aspects of the brain or brainstem, could also be due to the same lesion. Let's follow Occam's razor and assume that the simplest explanation is the correct explanation, and all of her signs and symptoms are due to a single lesion involving the right parietal and, possibly, occipital lobes.

WHAT IS THE DIFFERENTIAL DIAGNOSIS?

Her syndromic diagnosis *is* a hyperacute onset of a right, nondominant parietal syndrome.

WHAT IS THE DIFFERENTIAL DIAGNOSIS?

The etiologic diagnosis includes vascular events and seizure. Since there is no description of seizure-like activity, then a vascular event (ischemic or hemorrhagic) is most likely.

CLINICAL COURSE AND ADDITIONAL INFORMATION

Her initial head imaging showed a hemorrhage in the right parieto-occipital lobes (Figure 18.1).

Her imaging is consistent with the hyperacute onset of her symptoms. Typically, an intracerebral hemorrhage causes symptoms within seconds to minutes of onset. So far, her imaging

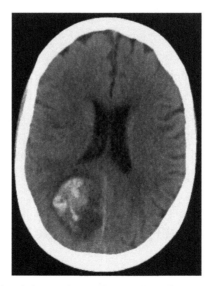

Figure 18.1. CT head shows a hemorrhage in the right parieto-occipital lobes.

fits her clinical syndrome. Is this the end diagnosis? It's a safe bet, since I included this case, that we have a bit more work to do before getting to the final diagnosis. Were there any changes to her imaging after her examination worsened? Could the pace or progression of her symptoms be a clue to the underlying cause of her hemorrhage? Let's look at her subsequent imaging in Figure 18.2, obtained in the setting of her clinical deterioration.

Her imaging worsened, corresponding to her deteriorating clinical status. It could be that her progressively worsening neurologic exam is simply a sequela of severe intracerebral hemorrhage. We do frequently see either extension of prior hemorrhage or clinical worsening due to other medical illness in the hospital, which can cause a patient's neurologic exam to worsen after the initial injury.

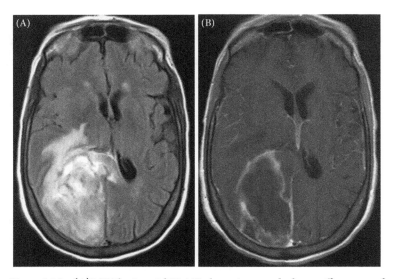

Figure 18.2. (**A**) MRI brain axial FLAIR shows increased edema, effacement of the occipital horn of the lateral ventricle, and midline shift. (**B**) MRI brain T1 post-contrast shows an irregular contrast-enhancing border.

However, I am intentionally including this case to highlight a critical point. Let's review the history again.

Her condition deteriorated over the next several days. She developed plegia of her left arm and leg followed by the left lower face. She eventually became unarousable to stimuli.

That is a severe and quick neurologic decline. What is the pace of her decline? She is worsening over hours to days. This fits within an acute pace of disease, as discussed earlier. How do we reconcile this with her initial hyperacute onset of symptoms? What if the same underlying etiology is presenting with two simultaneous syndromes—both a hyperacute onset and then acute progressive worsening? We already discussed, and then saw on her imaging, that her hyperacute onset was consistent with a vascular event, in this case an intracerebral hemorrhage. What are the possible etiologies of an acute onset of a cerebral syndrome with worsening clinical and radiographic progression? Since we have a large lesion on our imaging, we can safely exclude toxic or metabolic conditions. We are left with inflammatory or infectious conditions.

WHAT IS THE CONTEXT?

Our patient is a 66-year-old immunosuppressed woman with a history of stem cell transplant who initially presented with a cough and fever. In this context, infection seems like a more likely etiology of acute neurologic syndrome due to a rapidly enlarging mass lesion than an inflammatory disorder. At this point, it would be just guessing to name a pathogen without obtaining a biopsy.

CONCLUSION

Due to the rapid nature of her decline, she underwent biopsy of one of the masses seen in her lungs (Figure 18.3) as well as her brain.

Her biopsies showed invasive mucormycosis in the lung and brain. Mucormycosis is a fungus found in the environment that causes rare, but often fatal, infections in immunocompromised individuals. Infected hosts breathe spores from the environment that germinate into hyphae in the alveoli. Mucormycosis is angioinvasive and has a strong tropism for blood vessels. Her intracerebral hemorrhage was due to hematogenous seeding of mucormycosis from the lungs to the brain. This caused a CNS infection and secondary intracerebral hemorrhage. Unfortunately, the infection was ultimately fatal.

This case highlights the limitations, but also the power, of *pace*. On the one hand, her initial pace of onset was hyperacute. At first

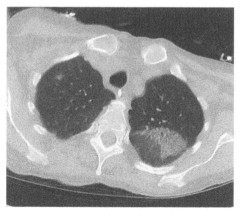

Figure 18.3. CT chest shows mass-like opacities in the apex of the left lung as well as scattered nodular opacities suggestive of fungal multifocal pneumonia.

glance, we would not have expected that to have been caused by an invasive fungal infection of the brain. However, her initial syndrome was caused by a hemorrhage, so in that sense the case did follow the rules established in the introductory chapter. She subsequently worsened over an acute time scale, which correspondingly was caused by a CNS infection. That again follows the rules. The methods of following *pace* and *localization* are frequently limited by the fact that the primary *pathologic diagnosis* might present with multiple different *paces* depending on its secondary effects. In some cases, that can be a hindrance to making the correct diagnosis. However, in some instances, such as this case, focusing on the multiple distinct *paces* of disease can actually lead to the pathologic diagnosis.

Chapter 19

A man with dyspnea and orthopnea

A 79-year-old man presented to the hospital with dyspnea and orthopnea over the past several weeks. He had a complex medical history of Waldenstrom's macroglobulinemia, amyloidosis, prostate cancer, melanoma, and squamous cell carcinoma. After admission to the hospital, he described having had weakness in his bilateral upper extremities. On further questioning, he stated that he initially developed weakness in his right arm approximately 2 months prior to being admitted to the hospital. He had difficulties with fine coordination of the right hand as well as raising the arm to brush his teeth or wash his hair. Several weeks later he developed weakness in his left arm. This was more severe than the right arm, to the point at which he could barely lift his left arm over his head. He denied any sensory changes. He had no difficulty walking, and he had no imbalance. There were no bowel or bladder changes. He denied any problems with his vision, including diplopia, nor did he have any symptoms of dysphagia or dysarthria. He denied any fluctuations in his symptoms or fatigability. He denied muscle pain or cramps.

Although it is tempting to go down the rabbit hole of his multiple malignancies and how they could be contributing to his symptoms, let's focus on localization first before generating diagnostic hypotheses.

What clues in the history help us target our exam? Often the "pertinent negatives" are more helpful in localizing the lesion or targeting our neurologic exam than the "pertinent positives." An arm can be weak for any reason from the muscle belly all the way up to the cortex and anywhere in between. However, the lack of many associated symptoms (sensory changes, fatigability, bowel/bladder symptoms) will have a very high yield for identifying the potential source of the problem.

On examination, he was well-appearing and in good spirits. Mental status and cranial nerve examinations were normal, most notable for normal extraocular movements and facial strength, no dysarthria, normal palate movement, and full tongue strength. He had no fasciculations or percussion myotonia. Muscle bulk and tone were mildly decreased in both upper extremities. Neck flexion was mildly weak. His right arm was mildly weak both proximally and distally: shoulder abduction 4/5, elbow flexion 4+/5, elbow extension 4−/5, wrist flexion and extension 4/5, finger flexion 4/5, finger extension 4−/5, thumb abduction 4−/5, and finger abduction 4−/5. His left arm strength was more variably affected: shoulder abduction 1/5, elbow flexion 2/5, elbow extension 4/5, wrist flexion 5/5, wrist extension 4/5, finger flexion 5/5, finger extension 4/5, thumb abduction 4/5, and finger abduction 4+/5. Strength in his lower extremities was normal. Sensory examination was normal, and reflexes were diminished in the upper extremities. Gait was normal, and he was able to tandem walk.

WHAT IS THE PACE?

His neurologic symptoms evolved over the course of several weeks to months, so the pace is subacute.

WHAT IS THE LOCALIZATION?

The first step is whether this is a lesion in the central or peripheral nervous system. He has a complete absence of any symptoms above the neck, making brain or brainstem involvement unlikely given the widespread degree of motor involvement. Although it is theoretically possible he could have multiple lesions in the motor cortex bilaterally sparing the face and lower extremities as well as sensation, this seems unlikely. In addition, the pattern of his weakness is not what we could consider an "upper motor neuron pattern." There is variable weakness throughout both extremities, particularly in his left arm. Some actions tested are strikingly normal, whereas the adjacent muscle is strikingly weak. Muscle tone and muscle stretch reflexes were diminished.

What constitutes an "upper motor neuron pattern" of weakness is worth discussing. Although the term is used almost ubiquitously in clinical practice and in textbooks, it is poorly understood. In fact, one of the purported key features of upper motor neuron weakness, upper extremity extensor weakness out of proportion to flexor weakness (and vice versa in the lower extremities), is likely false. The upper extremity extensor muscles generate less force than flexors in normal individuals. Thus, the examiner is more likely to judge an extensor muscle as weak than a flexor muscle based on the examiner's own strength. This pattern of preferential weakness of agonist/antagonist pairs, sometimes also referred to as a "pyramidal pattern" of weakness, is likely an illusion created by our non-objective bedside exam testing. More reliable features of upper versus lower motor neuron weakness include examination of muscle tone, muscle bulk, reflexes, and the presence or absence of fasciculations. In addition, upper motor neuron lesions tend to cause slowness in addition to weakness of movements, whereas speed of movements is relatively preserved even when there is weakness in lower motor neuron injuries.

Could the lesion be in the spinal cord? We would still expect a lesion in the spinal cord to have upper motor neuron signs on examination. Those axons, whose cell bodies reside in the motor cortex, comprise the lateral corticospinal tracts contralateral to their cortical origin. Although there are instances in which a spinal cord lesion may *not* show upper motor neuron signs, this doesn't rule out a spinal cord lesion completely. Because both upper extremities are involved, a spinal cord lesion would have to be large enough to affect both lateral corticospinal tracts while somehow sparing all leg motor function, sensation, and bowel and bladder function. Alternatively, there would have to be multiple small lesions somehow only involving the motor fibers traveling to the upper extremities. Both of these options seem unlikely. The lesion must therefore be in the peripheral nervous system.

Since he has complete preservation of sensation, we can substantially narrow down the localization within the peripheral nervous system. We can get a pure motor syndrome from a lesion at the level of the muscle or neuromuscular junction. Perhaps more complicated, but we could also get a lesion selective to the peripheral motor nerves. Since sensation is normal, this couldn't be a "straightforward" peripheral neuropathy as those diseases (such as diabetic peripheral neuropathy) don't selectively target motor nerve fibers.

Let's now go back to our history and look for those "pertinent negatives." If this were a myopathy, we might expect that he would have muscle cramping or pain. These are lacking. In addition, many myopathies, depending on the type, may have a pattern, such as proximal-greater-than-distal involvement or vice versa. These are both absent. If this were a neuromuscular junction problem such as myasthenia gravis, we might expect to obtain a history of fluctuations in severity of his symptoms or fatigability. Both of these are absent. Thus, of our three possible peripheral nervous system possible localizations (muscle, neuromuscular junction, or lower motor nerves), lower motor nerves seem the most likely to be affected.

Before proceeding, there is one large caveat to this discussion. Often our history and examination can only get us so far in terms of localization. Even the world's foremost experts in neuromuscular disorders frequently can't make a diagnosis without the use of an electromyogram and nerve conduction studies (EMG/NCS). This is why an EMG/NCS is frequently referred to as an extension of the neurologic exam. In clinical practice, an EMG/NCS is often critical in correctly localizing the lesion.

WHAT IS THE SYNDROMIC DIAGNOSIS?

We now know this is a subacute disorder that affects the peripheral nervous system at the level of the lower motor nerves, neuromuscular junction, or muscle. Of those options, the "pertinent negatives" in our history lead us away from a neuromuscular junction or muscle process. Our final syndromic hypothesis, which we will test with an EMG/NCS, is that he has a subacute disorder primarily involving the lower motor nerves.

His EMG/NCS helped confirm the localization we suspected. It showed active denervation in multiple nerves and myotomes throughout the cervical region. He had mildly prolonged F-wave latency (a supramaximal stimulation of a nerve that causes a muscle action potential to propagate antidromically "up" a nerve back to the spinal cord that then bounces back "down" the nerve and can be recorded). He also had conduction block of the compound muscle action potential. These both indicate dysfunction of the motor nerve fibers.

WHAT IS THE ETIOLOGIC DIAGNOSIS?

This is a subacute disorder, so our etiologic differential diagnosis includes autoimmune, infectious, and malignant diseases in addition to drugs/toxins/metabolic disorders. In this case, based on the sporadic, asymmetric involvement, some pathologic diagnoses are less likely. For example, it would be unlikely for an infectious process to somehow cause severe, patchy damages exclusively to the motor nerve fibers within the peripheral nerves while sparing sensory nerve fibers. Likewise, direct invasion of a neoplastic process only into certain parts of peripheral nerves is highly unlikely. We might also assume that a widespread metabolic or toxic process shouldn't be restricted to certain parts of nerves or regions of the body. Thus, we are left with the most likely process being an autoimmune disorder exclusively of the lower motor nerves. If you type this into your search engine of choice, you will find the ultimate pathologic diagnosis.

CONCLUSION

Multifocal motor neuropathy (MMN) is a pure motor neuropathy that typically presents with subacute onset of asymmetric motor deficits. Patients with MMN frequently have anti-ganglioside antibodies. Gangliosides are abundantly present on the surface of myelin and nodes of Ranvier in the peripheral nervous system. Although MMN is rare, it is a critical diagnostic consideration in the work-up of amyotrophic lateral sclerosis (ALS). It can present similarly (although the pace tends to be faster), but it is easily treatable in comparison to ALS.

BONUS QUESTION: CAN WE EXPLAIN HIS DYSPNEA AND ORTHOPNEA?

Go all the way back to the initial history. He was admitted to the hospital originally for dyspnea and orthopnea. Can this potentially be explained by MMN? Just like the motor nerves in his upper extremities are affected, the motor nerves that innervate the respiratory muscles can also be affected. Look at Figure 19.1 to see why he becomes short of breath when he lies down.

He has an elevated left hemi-diaphragm that worsens with inspiration. The left hemi-diaphragm is paretic. This is due to dysfunction of the phrenic nerve due to multifocal motor neuropathy. During inspiration, the diaphragm contracts and move downwards. When he is standing, gravity helps assist this muscle action. When he lies down, the diaphragm loses its gravity assistance and his symptoms worsen.

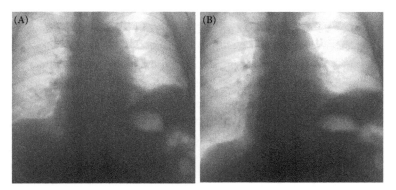

Figure 19.1. Chest radiograph (**A**) during exhalation and (**B**) during inhalation. On inspiration, the abnormally elevated left hemi-diaphragm does not move.

Chapter 20

A man with difficulty walking and spasms in his legs

A 31-year-old man with a history of adrenal insufficiency presented for evaluation of difficulty walking. He initially noted difficulty with balance and bilateral leg weakness while running. However, this progressed over the course of several months to the point at which he could notice symptoms even at rest. Within a year of symptom onset, he required a cane to walk, and he had suffered several falls. His legs felt very stiff, and he had difficulty sleeping due to jerking and spasms in his legs. He subsequently developed urinary urgency as well as hesitancy. In addition, he noted new onset of erectile dysfunction as well as worsening constipation. He was a physician, and he denied any cognitive difficulties at work. With regards to his past medical history, his diagnosis of adrenal insufficiency was made while he was in high school after he went into severe shock after a simple viral illness. He also had diffuse new onset of skin hyperpigmentation during the preceding winter months.

As always, begin to formulate your hypothesis regarding the localization in the history. Difficulty walking could be due to numerous conditions, and the history frequently provides critical context that shapes the neurologic exam. Associated symptoms are important clues. For some cases, the clinical context is tantalizing from the get-go. His adrenal dysfunction may play a role in our final etiologic diagnosis, but try to be patient and work through the steps of pace and localization before guessing at specific disorders.

On examination, he was well-appearing with a tan appearance. Mental status and cranial nerve examinations were normal. Strength in his upper extremities was normal. Tone was mildly increased in the bilateral lower extremities. He had symmetric, mild weakness (4 to 4– at worst) in both legs both proximally and distally. His reflexes were elevated in the lower extremities, and both of his toes were mute (neither up-going nor down-going). Vibratory sensation was absent at the toes, diminished at the ankles, and present at the knees. Proprioception was also impaired, and he had a positive Romberg test. He walked with a cane and had a bilateral mild foot drop. An MRI of his brain and spinal cord was normal.

WHAT IS THE PACE?

His symptoms progressed over months to years, which is consistent with a chronic pace of illness.

WHAT IS THE LOCALIZATION?

His examination is most notable for a spastic paraparesis: He has mild weakness and increased tone/hyperreflexia in the bilateral lower extremities. As discussed in other cases, his increased tone and reflexes are upper motor neuron signs that point to a lesion within the central nervous system. Theoretically, this could localize anywhere along the corticospinal tracts, beginning in the bilateral motor cortices all the way down to its termination on the lower motor neurons that exit the cord to carry motor signals to the muscles. Since the lower extremities map medially within the motor homunculus, a single lesion could cause bilateral lower extremity symptoms. There are certain instances in which this is possible (such as a large parasagittal meningioma). A brainstem process seems less likely given the lack of cranial nerve abnormalities, and a cervical cord lesion also seems less likely due to lack of upper extremity involvement. Let's use other aspects of his history to help more definitively localize the lesion.

In addition to his motor dysfunction, he also has prominent urinary, sexual, and bowel dysfunction. These systems rely on both parasympathetic and sympathetic inputs. For example, normal micturition requires a balance of sympathetic and parasympathetic pathways between the sacral and pontine micturition centers (Figure 20.1). All of these actions can be mediated by cortical inhibition, but in a person without evidence of cortical dysfunction, then the localization for bowel, bladder, and sexual dysfunction is most likely a spinal cord injury. Since his motor symptoms apparently spare the upper extremities, the only unifying localization for these symptoms could be the thoracic spinal cord (despite his normal MRI).

He also has sensory loss in his bilateral lower extremities. Interestingly, his symptoms are bilateral and seem length-dependent: Vibration is absent at the toes, diminished at the ankles, and normal at the knees. Does his pattern of sensory loss localize to the spinal cord? We already suspect a spinal cord localization, and a

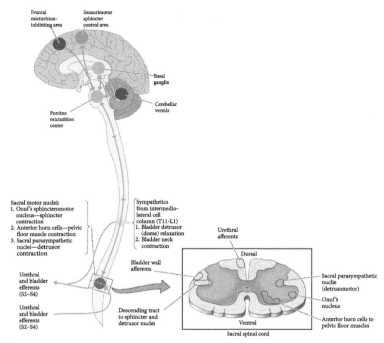

Figure 20.1. Illustration depicting the control of micturition. Normal micturition requires a balance between sympathetic and parasympathetic input, which is ultimately mediated by the pontine micturition center and higher cortical input. *Reproduced by permission from Hal Blumenfeld, Neuroanatomy through Clinical Cases (New York, New York: Oxford University Press, 2018), 294.*

spinal cord lesion can most surely cause sensory loss. However, his symptoms are length-dependent. The distal lower extremities are more affected than the proximal lower extremities. This is a typical pattern for a peripheral polyneuropathy.

How do we put this all together? Is his lesion a myelopathy or a myeloneuropathy (a myelopathy *and* a peripheral neuropathy)? As discussed previously, the neurologic exam, although a powerful tool, is not always definitive. In this case, a nerve conduction study showed damage to the peripheral nerves, confirming their involvement.

WHAT IS THE SYNDROMIC DIAGNOSIS?

He presents with a chronic myeloneuropathy. Don't be swayed by the normal imaging of his spine! The clinical syndrome doesn't fit any other possible localization.

WHAT IS THE ETIOLOGIC DIAGNOSIS?

Since this is a chronic disease, we can narrow down the etiologic diagnosis to either a genetic, neurodegenerative, neoplastic, or toxic/metabolic phenomenon. We can immediately rule out a slow-growing neoplasm given his normal imaging of the brain and spinal cord. We are then left with either a genetic, neurodegenerative, or toxic/metabolic process. Presumably any of these disorders might require blood or spinal fluid testing to identify, and if you were to put "chronic myeloneuropathy" into a search engine, you would be rewarded with a long list of exotic and fascinating diseases. In instances in which the syndromic diagnosis doesn't have a readily apparent cause, and the possible etiologic diagnoses are rare and variable, we need to rely on the context (if available) to help us target our testing.

His history is notable for adrenal insufficiency. Here we can invoke Occam's razor. As discussed in the introduction, Occam's razor tends to be more reliable in younger patients who are less likely to have multiple illnesses. This is particularly true if they have a relatively uncommon preexisting illness. The likelihood that his uncommon neurologic syndrome is linked to his uncommon adrenal insufficiency is high. Now all we need to do is check to see if there is a single unifying diagnosis that links his adrenal insufficiency to myeloneuropathy.

Whereas the work-up for an individual with a chronic myeloneuropathy without clinical context relies on the "shotgun" method of laboratory testing, the work-up for an individual with adrenal insufficiency and myeloneuropathy is quite straightforward. I encourage you to input those terms into your search engine of choice, and you will find the pathologic diagnosis.

CONCLUSION

Adrenomyeloneuropathy is an X-linked inherited condition due to a genetic mutation in the *ABCD1* gene. Individuals with a pathogenic mutation in the *ABCD1* gene typically present in childhood with a neurologic syndrome called adrenoleukodystrophy or in young adulthood with adrenomyeloneuropathy. These are not distinct disorders, and individuals with adrenomyeloneuropathy can have brain involvement. The *ABCD1* gene encodes for a protein involved in the transport of very-long-chain fatty acids into peroxisomes. Pathogenic mutations in adrenomyeloneuropathy cause low levels of this protein; this leads to elevated levels of very-long-chain fatty acids and the clinical phenotype.

Chapter 21

A woman with recurrent episodes of confusion and stiffness

A 19-year-old woman presented for evaluation of stereotyped episodes of confusion. She (and her mother) described the episodes, which began 1 month prior, as follows: She developed sudden onset of stiffness in her extremities and her eyes would roll back into her head. She would retain consciousness during the episodes, but she appeared drowsy and slower to answer questions. The episodes would last for only a few minutes. It would take her approximately 30 to 60 minutes after an episode to feel back to her baseline. Her mother checked her pulse during one of these attacks and noted it seemed to be slow. In total, she had approximately five of these episodes over a month. Concurrent with these episodes she noted decreased dexterity in her left hand that was present even in between the episodes. In addition to these episodes, she had a history of headaches, which had worsened in frequency and intensity over the past year. She described the headaches as holocephalic, throbbing, and associated with nausea.

She appears to have two distinct clinical syndromes. One is manifest by stereotypical episodes of transient neurologic dysfunction. However, in the background is what appears to be more fixed deficits.

We will need to determine whether these distinct clinical syndromes are secondary to the same underlying diagnosis or if they are disparate disorders. So far, her history has not significantly helped us to focus our neurologic exam. The localization and differential diagnosis remain quite broad.

Her neurologic examination, performed when she was at her baseline between episodes, revealed a normal mental status. There was mild blurring of the optic discs bilaterally. Otherwise, the rest of her cranial nerve examination was normal. Motor testing was normal with the exception of mild weakness of the intrinsic muscles of the left hand. Sensory examination was normal. Her reflexes were brisk with spread in the lower extremities and up-going toes bilaterally. She had no ataxia, and her gait was normal.

WHAT IS THE PACE?

She presents with sudden onset of neurologic symptoms lasting minutes, which is consistent with a hyperacute pace of disease. However, she also noted static weakness of her hand as well as worsening headaches. This could indicate a superimposed process that, by history, seems to have a chronic pace of disease.

WHAT IS THE LOCALIZATION?

We don't have much here to help us localize the lesion. Let's start with the findings on her examination.

She has mild weakness in her left hand and hyperreflexia in her bilateral lower extremities. This doesn't tell us too much besides the fact that she has evidence of upper motor neuron involvement of the corticospinal tracts (hyperreflexia), which indicates the lesion is in the central nervous system. However, it could involve anywhere along the length of the corticospinal tracts.

The only other finding on her exam is some mild blurring of her optic discs bilaterally. This is frequently due to papilledema, swelling of the optic discs due to increased intracranial pressure (ICP). Her new headaches could also be due to elevated ICP. However, these signs and symptoms do not help us localize further within the central nervous system.

Lastly, even the periodic attacks she is having do not provide much value in terms of localization. The most notable feature is that she has decreased level of arousal, but, as discussed in other cases, this has broad localization from the brainstem to the cortices.

WHAT IS THE SYNDROMIC DIAGNOSIS?

She presents with hyperacute onset of poorly localizing transient neurologic deficits. Since she has evidence of increased ICP, as evident by the blurring of the optic discs and episodic confusion, we might expect a lesion somewhere within the calvarium, but we cannot be more specific than that. We also have additional static, possibly chronic, symptoms of impaired left-handed dexterity.

WHAT IS THE ETIOLOGIC DIAGNOSIS?

Our *etiologic* differential diagnosis of hyperacute-onset transient neurologic symptoms includes stroke, seizure, headache, trauma, structural, and toxic/metabolic disorders. There is no history of trauma, and there is no evidence of toxin exposure or metabolic disarray. Thus, we are left with stroke, seizure, structural, and headache disorders. Although she has headaches, that does not explain her fixed left-hand weakness or hyperreflexia. Is this a vascular event or a seizure? These episodes are stereotyped and last only a few minutes, which fits nicely with seizure. If these events are seizures, we still expect to see a focal, space-occupying lesion on imaging to explain her papilledema, headaches, and left-hand weakness.

ADDITIONAL INFORMATION

Her MRI, depicted in Figure 21.1, showed a type I Chiari malformation, which is a congenital dysgenesis associated with a constellation of abnormalities, such as cerebellar tonsillar herniation, displacement of the lower brainstem, and syringomyelia. Chiari malformations, although not uncommonly seen on imaging, may be incidental findings, and many patients are often asymptomatic. The degree of symptom associated with a Chiari malformation an individual experiences tends to be associated with the degree of impairment of normal CSF flow. As depicted in Figure 21.1C, her phase-contrast MRI showed impaired CSF flow around the foramen magnum as well as hydrocephalus and a large syringomyelia.

Thus far, I have intentionally chosen cases that have not relied as heavily on imaging to generate the differential diagnosis. However, in practice, imaging or other ancillary testing is very frequently used in more than just an adjunct role to make a diagnosis. However, even when an imaging abnormality is discovered, we can't state definitively that the findings seen on MRI are the cause of the patient's symptoms without applying our syndromic diagnosis.

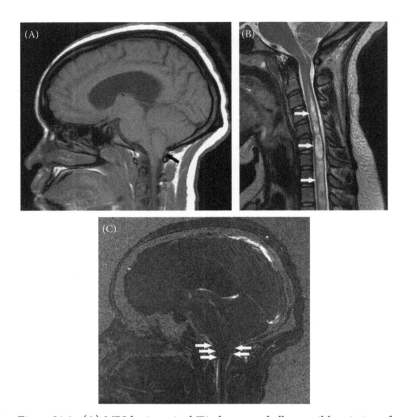

Figure 21.1. (**A**) MRI brain sagittal T1 shows cerebellar tonsil herniation of 6 mm past the foramen magnum (*arrow*). The third and fourth ventricles are mildly enlarged, consistent with hydrocephalus. (**B**) MRI sagittal cervical spine T2 demonstrates an extensive syringomyelia extending throughout the cervical and thoracic spine (*arrows*). (**C**) MRI brain cine sequence shows poor CSF flow across the foramen magnum anterior to the brainstem and posterior to the cerebellar tonsils (*arrows*).

Are the features seen on her MRI acute on chronic? By history and exam, she had new headaches and findings of elevated ICP on exam. In addition, she had new weakness in her left hand. All of these signs and symptoms indicate an evolving process and raise our

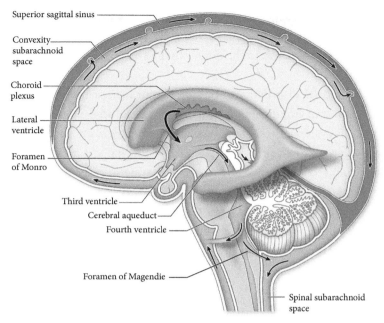

Superior sagittal sinus

Convexity subarachnoid space

Choroid plexus

Lateral ventricle

Foramen of Monro

Third ventricle

Cerebral aqueduct

Fourth ventricle

Foramen of Magendie

Spinal subarachnoid space

Figure 21.2. Diagram of CSF flow. The choroid plexus produces spinal fluid, which flows out of the calvarium by way of the third ventricle through the cerebral aqueduct and fourth ventricle. Spinal fluid then circulates around the spinal cord and roots, returning to the cerebral convexity, and is reabsorbed by arachnoid granulations. *Republished with permission of McGraw Hill LLC, from Adams and Victor's Principles of Neurology, Ropper, Allan H., Martin A. Samuels, Joshua P. Klein, and Sashank Prasad, 11th edition, 2019; permission conveyed through Copyright Clearance Center, Inc.*

suspicion that her imaging findings are the cause of her symptoms. Could her imaging findings also explain her transient episodes?

CONCLUSION

I mentioned in the introduction that the cases wouldn't focus on structural (non-oncologic compressive lesions) disorders.

Structural disorders can cause disruptions in CSF flow, either too much (such as a CSF leak) or too little (such as in this case), as well as direct damage to the nerves themselves. Figure 21.2 depicts CSF flow.

Structural disorders can be due to extrinsic or intrinsic compression and impingement on parts of the central or peripheral nervous system. These disorders can present with any pace. There are a variety of etiologies that can cause mechanical compression of various components of the nervous system, such as systemic malignancy, degenerative spine disease, or trauma. Even though these disorders have not been the focus of our other cases, they are equally important to consider when a patient presents with a neurologic syndrome. In these cases when imaging reveals a possible structural disorder, the role of the neurologist is to determine whether the abnormality seen on imaging can cause the clinical syndrome, or if further investigation for alternative diagnoses needs to be pursued. In practice, imaging frequently reveals structural abnormalities, but in many cases, these structural abnormalities are incidental.

In this case, her symptoms fully resolved after decompression of her Chiari malformation. In addition, her EEG did not show any evidence of seizures. Given the improvement after decompression, the suspected *pathologic diagnosis* was that her Chiari malformation led to impaired CSF flow around the foramen magnum. She then developed transient episodes of markedly elevated ICP spikes, which manifested as her transient confusional episodes. Descriptions of similar episodes of altered mental status have been seen in other disorders that can cause dramatic spikes of elevated ICP, such as in leptomeningeal malignancies.

Chapter 22

A man who could only see half of La Sagrada Familia

A 30-year-old right-handed man developed headache and photophobia. He initially attributed these symptoms to difficulty sleeping, which was also new to him. He felt well enough that he went on vacation several weeks later. However, while traveling, he became more confused. He forgot the names of his friends. When he tried to text his family about what he was experiencing, he couldn't unlock his phone with his PIN or spell words correctly. He had multiple generalized convulsions. Although he didn't remember much of the events during this time period, he was able to distinctly recall that when he looked out of his hotel room at La Sagrada Familia, the left side of the building appeared normal but the right side of it "just didn't make sense." He developed complex and formed visual hallucinations that he described as people who were not there or rainbows of color. Ultimately, his seizures worsened and his language abilities deteriorated, and he could no longer understand others or speak coherent sentences.

When we have the luxury of a detailed history, we have an advantage when performing the neurologic exam. We know the general location of the lesion based on the history alone. The role of the exam is two-fold. First, the exam should confirm our hypothesized localization based on the history. Second, the exam should also rule out other localizations or multifocal lesions. Be mindful not to fall into the trap of only performing a highly targeted exam that seeks to confirm your hypothesis rather than ruling out the null hypothesis.

The following examination occurred after he received treatment for his frequent seizures, which led to improvement in level of consciousness and language abilities.

On examination, he was alert and attentive. He had some difficulty with naming low-frequency objects, but otherwise language was normal. He described that faces in his right visual field (only) appeared abnormal and dysmorphic, "like a Picasso painting." He could not recognize familiar faces even though they did not look abnormal in the left visual field. He had dyschromatopsia, but only in the right visual field. For example, a slice of cake placed on his right side appeared green, but when it was moved to the left side it appeared its true color, pink. He was unable to identify simple shapes such as a circle or square by visual inspection alone. However, when allowed to trace objects with his finger, he was able to identify them correctly. Additionally, when asked to copy a figure such as a triangle on a page, he was unable to do so correctly, but when allowed to trace it first with his finger, he would be able to copy the figure. He was able to draw a triangle when verbally directed to do so (Figure 22.1). He was unable to perform simple calculations or tell time from a digital or analog clock. He could write, but when asked to read back a sentence he had written just minutes earlier, he was unable to read his own writing. He was an avid musician. However, even though he could listen to music and fully understand it, he lost the ability to play the piano. The rest of his

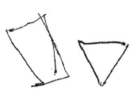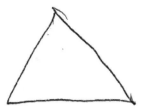

Figure 22.1. The patient's attempt to copy the figure (triangle) shown on the page. The figure on the *left* depicts a triangle drawn by the examiner and the patient's attempt at copying the figure. The large triangle on the *right* is his depiction of a triangle when given a verbal instruction to draw the geometric shape composed of three straight lines. He was subsequently unable to identify the figure he had just drawn.

neurologic exam, including cranial nerves, motor, sensory, and cerebellar testing, was all normal.

MRI brain with and without contrast was normal, and basic cerebrospinal fluid testing was within normal limits.

WHAT IS THE PACE?

His symptoms evolved over the course of weeks, which is consistent with a subacute pace of disease.

WHAT IS THE LOCALIZATION?

This is one of these cases where neurology is just cool. This is a man who can't count or even read what he writes, but he has the language ability of a healthy adult and can describe in detail what it is like to experience the world with such disabling symptoms! Let's go through his exam.

His visual processing was highly abnormal. Visual input is relayed from the retina via the optic nerves, tracts, and radiations to the primary visual cortex. However, wide networks of the brain are dedicated to processing these raw visual data. Although the initial or primary visual cortex receives raw visual data and can be thought of as your mind's projection of the surrounding environment, the brain requires large secondary visual cortical regions to make sense of the information it receives. The primary visual cortex initially registers data in 1s and 0s, whereas the secondary visual cortical regions assign meaning and context to the strings of 1s and 0s—face recognition, motion, symbols, etc.

There are three pathways that stream out from the primary visual cortex to other parts of the brain, termed the *what, where,* and *when* pathways (Figure 22.2). The *what* pathway assigns meaning to the raw data and helps us recognize faces, objects, and colors. The *where* pathway helps us with visuospatial orientation and tells us where things are in space. The *when* pathway helps us process motion and order. Information travels from the occipital lobe in a tangled, constant flow to various parts of the brain, and damage to any part of this extensive circuitry can have catastrophic effects.

He could write and speak, indicating his language ability was intact. He also could see primary visual data, but he could not process these raw visual data in a meaningful way; for example, he could not read. We refer to this as *alexia,* or the inability to read. Alexia is a type of agnosia, an inability to interpret or recognize a particular sensation, in this case a visual agnosia. This deficit is caused by damage to the *what* pathway. When writing is preserved, we refer to this constellation of findings as *alexia without agraphia.* Thus, he

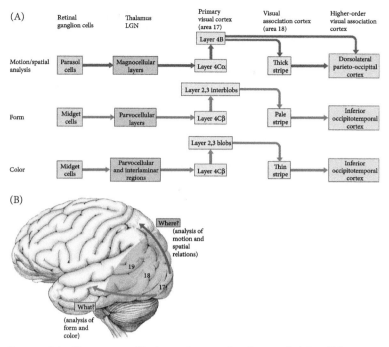

Figure 22.2. Illustration of higher-order visual pathways. (**A**) Parallel circuits encode information regarding motion, shape, and color. (**B**) The *what* and *where* pathways project from the primary visual cortex. *Reproduced by permission from Hal Blumenfeld, Neuroanatomy through Clinical Cases (New York, New York: Oxford University Press, 2018), 468.*

must have a deficit in the *what* pathway somewhere between the left primary visual cortex in the occipital lobe and the left parietal and temporal lobes.

In addition to his fascinating visual processing deficits, he could not perform basic elementary arithmetic. This is referred to as *acalculia*, the inability to perform math. This typically localizes to the left (dominant) angular gyrus. Music agnosia, although fascinating, is less well localized.

We have more than enough information to identify the localization. The lesion must be in the left (dominant) lobe affecting the *what* pathway as it travels from the primary visual cortex to the parietal and temporal lobes. Even though his MRI brain was normal (as noted earlier), we know there must be focal dysfunction in that region of the brain.

WHAT IS THE SYNDROMIC DIAGNOSIS?

He presents with a *syndromic* diagnosis of subacute onset of a focal cortical syndrome involving the left occipital, temporal, and parietal lobes.

WHAT IS THE ETIOLOGIC DIAGNOSIS?

Given the pace of his symptoms, the differential *etiologic diagnosis* is limited to infectious, inflammatory, and neoplastic disorders. It would be highly unlikely for him to have a metabolic process causing a progressive focal deficit, and there is nothing in the history to suggest infection, thus making those unlikely etiologies of his symptoms. His normal MRI makes cancer (and infection causing focal deficits) unlikely, since we would expect those to be more readily apparent on imaging. Thus, we are left an inflammatory disease as the most likely etiology of his presentation.

CONCLUSION

Even though his MRI and cerebrospinal fluid were both normal, he had a markedly abnormal positron emission tomography (PET)

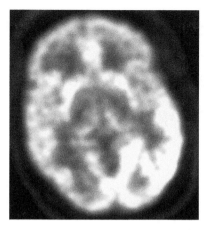

Figure 22.3. FDG-PET brain shows increased cortical metabolic activity in the left occipital, parietal, and temporal lobes.

brain that showed increased cortical metabolic activity in the left occipital, parietal, and temporal lobes (Figure 22.3). Several weeks after his spinal fluid was sent for testing, a positive result finally came back. He had anti-NMDA receptor encephalitis. This is an autoimmune disorder caused by autoantibodies that bind and block the neuronal cell-surface N-methyl-D-aspartate receptor. It can present with a wide range of phenotypes from relatively mild neuropsychiatric dysfunction all the way to coma and death. This presentation, with focal, predominantly visual deficits, is not common. He eventually recovered with appropriate treatment, and he had no neurologic deficits 1 year later.

Chapter 23

A boy who could no longer ride his bike

An 11-year-old boy initially presented for evaluation of nocturnal incontinence over the past year. He was born at full term, and there were no complications in the neonatal period. Prior to onset of his symptoms, he had no developmental delays. Since onset of his enuresis, his family noted that he tended to walk more slowly, and he was not very active. He used to enjoy riding his bike, but he began to complain to his parents it was difficult and stopped riding it. His initial evaluation uncovered spinal scoliosis and spina bifida occulta. He wore a brace for his scoliosis, but that did not improve his symptoms. His neurologic examination at that time was unremarkable. As part of the work-up for scoliosis, he had imaging of his brain (Figure 23.1) that revealed several abnormalities.

We are going to approach this case slightly differently. I am going to present some of the imaging prior to the rest of the history and neurologic exam, as that is the sequence of events that occurred.

The goal of this case is not to review the imaging. Suffice it to say, the differential at this time based solely on the imaging findings was an inflammatory or neoplastic process. For those of you with more

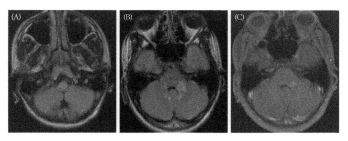

Figure 23.1. MRI brain axial FLAIR demonstrates abnormal signal changes in the (**A**) dorsal medulla and (**B**) left middle cerebellar peduncle. (**C**) MRI brain axial T1 post-contrast demonstrates contrast enhancement.

imaging expertise, you might be suspicious of demyelinating disorders such as multiple sclerosis. However, no definitive diagnosis was made of any condition on this MRI.

The following year he developed behavioral problems at school. However, he did well in classes and was on the A honor roll. Approximately 4 years after onset of his initial symptoms, at the age of 15, he began to experience dysphagia and dysarthria. He was diagnosed with severe obstructive sleep apnea. His dysphagia progressed to the point at which he needed a feeding tube. He was frequently hypothermic when seen in the clinic without evidence of infection. His performance at school declined significantly, but he was still on track to graduate.

Now, on examination several years into his clinical syndrome, he was hypothermic but well-appearing. He had mild dysarthria, but he was understandable and without cognitive deficits. He had a concomitant right hypertropia (skew deviation) and bilateral, direction-changing nystagmus. Muscle bulk and tone was normal, and his strength was full to confrontation. He had no abnormal movements. Reflexes were normal throughout, and his toes were down-going bilaterally. Sensation was intact throughout. He had dysmetria with finger-to-nose bilaterally, and his gait was cautious and wide-based.

WHAT IS THE PACE?

His symptoms developed over the span of several years, which is consistent with a chronic pace of illness.

WHAT IS THE LOCALIZATION?

Since I have already shown you an MRI, some of this shouldn't be too much of a surprise. He has dysarthria, a skew deviation, and bilateral, direction-changing nystagmus. These signs and symptoms are all consistent with a cerebellar lesion. In addition, he has significant dysphagia. If due to neurologic dysfunction, this would localize to nerves of the lower brainstem (medulla)—glossopharyngeal, vagus, or hypoglossal. Without a more detailed exam, we cannot determine exactly which nerves or nuclei might be affected. However, all of these findings are consistent with what we already saw on his imaging, that he has lesions on his MRI involving the medulla and cerebellum.

Does hypothermia have a localization? That is a more difficult question to answer. Hypothermia can be seen in certain conditions, such as hypothyroidism or hypoglycemia. He underwent extensive laboratory testing, which did not reveal any abnormalities. However, hypothermia can also be seen in lesions to the central nervous system. The hypothalamus is a key structure responsible for maintaining homeostasis within the body. Lesions of the hypothalamus can lead to thermoregulatory dysfunction, either hyperthermia or hypothermia. Lesions of the hypothalamus also frequently cause disorders of sleep and behavior and endocrine dysfunction. Additional injuries can also cause hypothermia, such as damage to the cervical spinal cord or medulla, which could impact the sympathetic output of the hypothalamus. Although we can't determine the localization definitively, the fact that he has such profound hypothermia indicates profound dysfunction to the thermoregulatory network.

CLINICAL COURSE AND ADDITIONAL INFORMATION

Unsurprisingly, the findings on his MRI 4 years after his initial imaging had progressed from what was seen previously (Figure 23.2).

WHAT IS THE SYNDROMIC DIAGNOSIS?

He presents with a chronic progression of a cerebellar and lower brainstem syndrome. Our syndromic diagnosis is relatively straightforward, especially with the assistance of his imaging findings.

WHAT IS THE ETIOLOGIC DIAGNOSIS?

Our differential of etiologic diagnoses includes malignancy, genetic disorders, neurodegenerative disease, and toxic/metabolic processes. In the absence of a history of exposure or laboratory

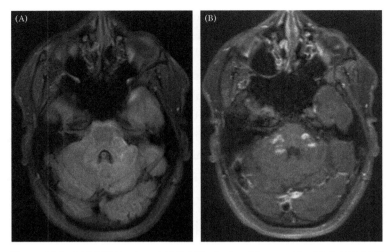

Figure 23.2. (**A**) MRI brain axial FLAIR obtained 4 years after his initial MRI shows more extensive signal change throughout the cerebellar peduncles, pons, and medulla. (**B**) MRI brain axial T1 post-contrast shows multiple enhancing lesions in the brainstem and middle cerebellar peduncles.

abnormalities, then toxic/metabolic processes are unlikely. Since he is a child, an inherited genetic disorder is far more likely than a neurodegenerative disease. Thus, we are left with either a neoplastic or genetic process. We might expect that if it were a neoplastic process, it would at least be a lower-grade malignancy due to the relatively slow progression over years. However, that would still not necessarily portend a "good" prognosis given the location of the lesions in the highly valuable brainstem.

CONCLUSION

This case is a good example of the limitations of the methods of *pace* and *localization*. In medicine, the full clinical syndrome is not always apparent in the initial stages of disease. When that occurs, it is impossible to make a diagnosis until time progresses and additional symptoms accrue (or symptoms remain stable). It is relatively easy, in hindsight after several years of symptoms, to suggest that this was a slowly progressing, relatively indolent process. However, at the time of initial presentation, when an 11-year-old child is found to have multiple large, mass-like lesions in his cerebellum and brainstem, we do not yet have that information. We offer little solace to the patient or his parents if we ask them to sit idly by while we wait for him to progress (or not). This balance between observation and intervention occasionally prevents us from using the concepts of *pace* and *localization*.

In this case, he underwent a biopsy of one of the enhancing lesions relatively soon after the lesions were discovered on his initial MRI. At the time (prior to years of progressive symptoms), the concern was for demyelinating diseases or malignancy. However, the pathology results revealed an atypical presentation of a rare genetic disorder, Alexander's disease.

Alexander's disease is caused by a mutation in glial fibrillary acidic protein (GFAP). It typically presents as a disease of infancy with progressive damage to the cerebral white matter. Pathology shows characteristic inclusions (called Rosenthal fibers) due to accumulation of the mutated intermediate filament protein. In the infantile form, there is widespread involvement of the cerebral white matter. However, Alexander's disease can rarely present with milder forms in late childhood and early adulthood. All forms are due to autosomal dominant mutations in GFAP, but they can have very distinct presentations, including cerebellar and brainstem syndromes.

In retrospect, our patient's syndrome followed the rules of pace and localization, but these rules were not helpful in identifying the diagnosis. In neurology, we typically cannot wait years for a clinical syndrome to develop or worsen to help us narrow down the differential from a severe autoimmune condition or cancer to a genetic disorder. Sometimes, we must act with incomplete data, and in those circumstances, *pace* and *localization* are no substitute for a tissue diagnosis.

Chapter 24

A woman with loss of consciousness while driving

A 36-year-old woman with a history of anxiety and panic disorder presented with recurrent spells of loss of consciousness. She had begun a new job several months prior and had been under significant psychological stress. She noted daily episodes of sudden, transient loss of consciousness. These episodes occurred with only momentary (seconds) warning. The episodes were unwitnessed and exclusively occurred in her car while she was driving, specifically while backing her car out of a parking spot. She believed that the duration was less than 1 to 2 minutes but could not be sure. She denied being confused after the episodes, and she denied any urinary incontinence or tongue biting. She ultimately presented for evaluation with neurology after she struck another car after losing consciousness while backing out of a parking space. At that time, she denied any other neurologic symptoms. Although she was under significant stress related to her work, she had no concerns regarding cognition. She denied any headache, vision changes, weakness, numbness, or gait difficulty.

> *At times a patient's chief complaint may not even sound like it is a neurologic condition. Especially given the context of this patient's significant stress, your first instinct might be to dismiss her symptoms as psychiatric, functional, or cardiac. Admittedly, this is an artificial exercise and the case is included in a book on unknown neurologic disorders, so she likely has a neurologic disorder. However, try to put yourself in the mindset of encountering this patient in the clinic or the emergency room. What about her history catches your attention that her presentation could hint at a neurologic disorder?*
>
> Her neurologic exam was normal. Her vital signs were normal in a seated and standing position. She had no orthostatic hypotension. However, she had several episodes of sinus brady-cardia while on telemetry monitoring that corresponded to turning her head to the left or right.

WHAT IS THE PACE?

The onset of her symptoms is seconds, which is consistent with a hyperacute pace.

WHAT IS THE LOCALIZATION?

This case is different than the others. She has a normal neurologic exam. Since her exam is normal, is this even a neurologic problem? How do we attempt to localize the lesion? Let's do this case slightly differently and come back to localization after we discuss the syn-dromic diagnosis.

WHAT IS THE SYNDROMIC DIAGNOSIS?

So far, we have only discussed neurologic disorders as the potential etiology of various presentations. However, patients may have a "non-neurologic" disorder that causes symptoms that can be construed as being neurologic in nature. For example, an elderly woman with severe osteoarthritis may have a chief complaint of gait difficulty. In addition, patients with psychiatric illness may present with neurologic manifestations of disease.

In the case of hyperacute loss of consciousness, in addition to the etiologies we have previously discussed, such as stroke, seizure, or metabolic abnormality, there is one other important etiology on the differential. Syncope is the loss of consciousness secondary to decreased cerebral perfusion, and as neurologists, we might mistakenly come to the conclusion that syncope is "non-neurologic" in origin. We typically look to the history to help us distinguish between syncope and other neurologic diagnoses, such as seizure or stroke. However, often the patient cannot provide the history if there are no witnesses. When a patient presents after an episode of loss of consciousness, we are frequently left asking the age-old question: Did they fall (syncope) or were they pushed (seizure)? Our ability to answer that question is usually most dependent on the history rather than any ancillary data collected after the fact.

In this case, does her presentation seem most consistent with a primary neurologic diagnosis, such as seizure or stroke? Are her symptoms more consistent with an alternative explanation, such as syncope or even panic attack? What are the salient features?

The episodes are brief and stereotyped, and she appears to have a warning prior to losing consciousness. In addition, she is not confused for a prolonged time period after the episode. This argues against a seizure in that we might expect her to have a post-ictal period if she had been having seizures. Stroke seems less likely given the stereotyped nature of the events and the fact that she has such profound loss of consciousness but is otherwise neurologically normal and makes a full recovery. The history fits well with syncope. In addition, she has episodes of sinus bradycardia, which could lead to syncope and be an important clue in making her final diagnosis.

Now we can return to localization. What is the localization of syncope, and how might we explain why she has syncope only when backing her car out of a parking spot? Can her syncope be secondary to a neurologic condition?

WHAT IS THE LOCALIZATION?

Syncope is not always due to a cardiac etiology. The nervous system exerts substantial control over heart rate and blood pressure. To understand syncope, we must first understand how the body regulates blood pressure.

$$Mean\ arterial\ pressure = (Cardiac\ output \times Systemic\ vascular\ resistance) + Central\ venous\ pressure$$

Since central venous pressure is typically close to 0 mmHg, we can simplify the formula as follows:

$$Mean\ arterial\ pressure = Cardiac\ output \times Systemic\ vascular\ resistance$$

For the purposes of this discussion, we will not discuss factors that lower mean arterial pressure (MAP) that are non-neurologic, such as decreased blood volume from hemorrhage. We will focus on the signals the nervous system receives regarding MAP (afferent input) and the mechanisms by which the nervous system responds to alternations in MAP (efferent output).

Figure 24.1 is a graphical representation of the following discussion. Baroreceptors in the carotid sinus (glossopharyngeal nerve) and aortic arch (vagus nerve) detect changes in arterial pressure and pulse pressure (systolic minus diastolic pressure). Of these two, the carotid sinus (located at the base of the internal carotid arteries) plays the more important role of detecting rapid, beat-to-beat changes in arterial pressure. These baroreceptors, with the carotid sinus being the dominant source of input for rapid changes in blood pressure, make up the afferent loop to the baroreflex. Of note, there are additional baroreceptors present in the atria of the heart and large pulmonary vessels that detect decreased blood volume. These receptors send their afferent signals to the endocrine system (such as hypothalamus) and lead to alterations in water and salt retention.

Nerves carrying information from the baroreceptors in the carotid sinus and aortic arch end in the medulla in the nucleus of the tractus solitarius (NTS). The NTS has multiple projections to the various efferent limbs of the baroreflex. First, the NTS sends signals to the dorsal motor nucleus of the vagus nerve. Vagal nerve fibers project to various components of the cardiac electrical conducting system, and increased vagal activity leads to decreased cardiac output via mechanisms such as decreased heart rate. Second, the NTS sends simultaneous signals to the intermediolateral cells of the thoracic spinal cord, which modulate systemic vascular resistance. Increased sympathetic outflow leads to vasoconstriction and an increase in systemic vascular resistance.

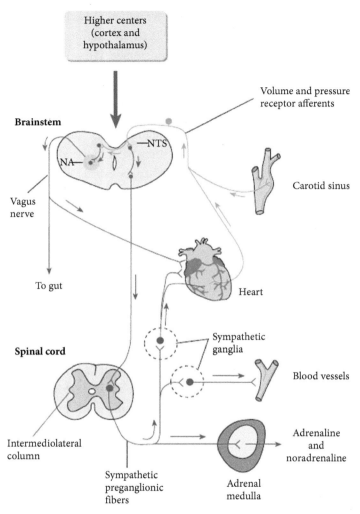

Figure 24.1. Schematic of the role of the autonomic nervous system in modulating the cardiovascular system. NA—nucleus ambiguous and NTS—nucleus tractus solitarius. *Reproduced by permission from Pocock, G., Christopher D. Richards, and David A. Richards, Human Physiology (Oxford, United Kingdom: Oxford University Press, 2013), 420.*

Although the anatomy is complicated, the end effect of barore-ceptor stimulation is quite simple. For example, a sudden decrease in blood pressure (such as what occurs going from sitting to standing) leads to decreased vagal activity and increased systemic vascular resistance. This causes an increase in heart rate and systemic vas-cular resistance to maintain a normal blood pressure. Conversely, a sudden increase in blood pressure leads to increased vagal activity, which causes decreased heart rate and decreased systemic vascular resistance.

We can summarize the preceding discussion as follows: Neurologic causes of syncope can involve lesions to either the afferent limb of the baroreflex (carotid sinus or aortic arch baroreceptors) or the efferent limb of the baroreflex (vagal or sym-pathetic outflow).

Now that we have discussed the localization of syncope in ge-neral, we can try to identify the localization of her specific lesion.

The history she provides is critical for localizing the lesion. If you need to, take a minute to review the case. She reports these episodes exclusively occurred while backing her car out of a parking spot. In addition, she had episodes of bradycardia when turning her head to the left or right. How can we explain this?

When she is backing her car out of a parking spot, she is turning her head to look over her shoulder. Presumably, this is causing brad-ycardia, just like what was seen on telemetry when she turned her head to the left or right. We can explain this using our knowledge of the baroreflex. When she turns her head she must be stimulating the baroreceptors in her carotid sinus, which is the afferent limb of the baroreflex. This leads to increased vagal activity to the heart and bradycardia as well as decreased sympathetic outflow and sys-temic vascular resistance. This must be the mechanism behind her syncope.

WHAT IS THE ETIOLOGIC DIAGNOSIS?

She presents with recurrent episodes of syncope. We suspect this is due to pathologic baroreflex activation of the carotid sinus, given that it only occurs when she turns her head to the left or right. Now we just need to take a close look at her carotid arteries to see if we can find an explanation as to why turning her head to one side or the other causes pathologic baroreflex activation.

CONCLUSION

A conventional angiogram (Figure 24.2) showed a left internal carotid artery dissection. In addition, she had a left vertebral artery

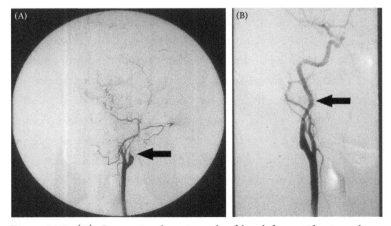

Figure 24.2. (**A**) Conventional angiograph of her left carotid artery shows tapering and occlusion (*arrow*) consistent with a right internal carotid artery dissection. (**B**) Conventional angiography of her right carotid artery shows the characteristic "beading" of fibromuscular dysplasia (*arrow*). *Images courtesy of Dr. David Paydarfar.*

dissection (not pictured) and a "beaded" appearance of the right internal carotid artery.

The etiologic diagnosis is intermittent carotid sinus dysfunction secondary to internal carotid artery dissection. Her multiple dissections as well as the "beaded" appearance of her right internal carotid artery are consistent with a pathologic diagnosis of fibromuscular dysplasia (FMD). The cause of FMD is unknown, but it is characterized as a non-artheromatous, non-inflammatory disease of the arteries that is almost exclusively seen in women. In her case, this led to arterial dissection, which presented with syncope due to damage of the afferent carotid baroreceptors.

For reference, other etiologies of pathologic carotid sinus syndromes include neoplasms exerting mechanical compression or arising within the carotid sinus, compression from the styloid process of the temporal bone, or other causes of intrinsic carotid disease such as atheromatous disease, vasculitis, or complications of carotid surgery.

Chapter 25

A man with painful feet

A 41-year-old man developed severe pain in both feet, which he described as sharp and icy. Approximately 18 months after his initial sensory symptoms, he developed dysphagia to solids and liquids. He had frequent emesis and early satiety, and he was only able to eat one small meal a day. Due to these symptoms, he lost over 30 lbs. His symptoms progressed, and his voice became hoarse and lower-pitched. He developed urinary hesitancy and severe constipation. He would frequently become light-headed when going from sitting to standing. Three years after the development of his symptoms, he began to lose strength in his hands, and he became weak in his lower extremities. At that point, he was walking with a cane, and his toes began to "curl." The pain that was initially in his feet subsequently spread to his legs and hands. Unfortunately, the pain was severe and refractory to multiple trials of different medications.

What are the salient features of his history that help us localize the lesion? Can we localize his GI symptoms and weight loss to his neurologic syndrome, or are these related but systemic manifestations of a systemic disease? If these symptoms are neurologic, how might that tie into his urinary dysfunction or orthostasis? A unique or unexpected symptom can be an important localizing clue. Take a minute to think about how neurologic dysfunction could lead to these other symptoms. We can use those clues to help focus our exam.

On examination, he was cachectic and ill-appearing. Mental status and cranial nerve examination was normal except for a mildly dysphonic voice. He was weak in his bilateral upper and lower extremities, worse distally in the hands and feet compared to proximally, and better than anti-gravity throughout. He had high-arched feet bilaterally, and he had wasting of the intrinsic muscles of his hands and feet (Figure 25.1). There were

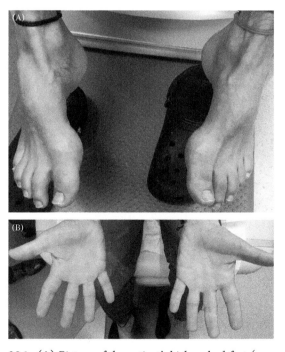

Figure 25.1. (**A**) Picture of the patient's high-arched feet (pes cavus). When due to a neurologic disorder, this is thought to be related to preferential weakness in agonist/antagonist pairs. (**B**) Picture of the patient's hands showing muscle wasting of the thenar and hypothenar eminences.

fasciculations in his forearms and legs. Reflexes were barely detectable in the upper extremities and absent in the lower extremities, and his plantar reflex was mute. Pinprick sensation was absent up to the thighs bilaterally in the lower extremities and the elbows in the bilateral upper extremities. Proprioception was absent in the toes and fingers. He had a positive Romberg test. He walked with a cane and had a prominent steppage gait.

WHAT IS THE PACE?

His symptoms evolved over years without any events that occurred on a faster time scale, so the pace is chronic.

WHAT IS THE LOCALIZATION?

First, we need to determine if this is a central or a peripheral process. Based on the history, his initial symptoms were a sharp and icy pain in his feet, which could be consistent with a peripheral length-dependent neuropathy. However, he also has prominent and early dysphagia, bowel, and bladder symptoms. At first glance, this could seem like a clue toward a lesion in the CNS such as the brainstem or spinal cord. However, his exam shows a clear "stocking-glove" distribution of sensory and motor dysfunction as well as absent reflexes and fasciculations (spontaneous lower motor neuron action potentials, which can be caused by damage or irritation to the cell membrane). All of these features point to a disorder of the peripheral nervous system.

His early dysphagia, bowel, and bladder symptoms don't seem to fit with a typical length-dependent neuropathy (such as the neuropathy caused by longstanding uncontrolled diabetes). All of these processes—digestion, bowel and bladder control, as well as blood pressure—are regulated by the autonomic nervous system (ANS). Remember, the ANS typically comprises preganglionic neurons (cell body located in the CNS) and postganglionic neurons (cell body located in the PNS). The nerves to those various organs aren't particularly lengthy.

When encountering a patient for the first time years into an illness, the current symptoms and examination may falsely localize the syndrome that was apparent at the onset of disease. For example, a patient with longstanding, untreated mononeuritis multiplex may have an examination consistent with a length-dependent polyneuropathy solely because of the accumulated burden of nerves involved over time. Because he has had symptoms for a few years, let's focus on just the early symptoms for our localization.

Given the presence of both a length-dependent sensory neuropathy and autonomic neuropathy, the localization is unlikely to be based on the typical geographic divisions of the peripheral nervous system (radiculopathy, plexopathy, neuropathy, etc.). However, we can also localize the lesion based on the subset of neurons or fibers (such as the anterior horn cells in ALS). With that clue in mind, can we localize his early satiety, bowel and bladder dysfunction, and orthostasis to a similar subset of neurons as those causing his sensory symptoms?

Table 25.1 provides a broad overview of the different types of nerve fibers. Some peripheral nerve fibers have a small diameter whereas others have a large diameter. Not all fibers are myelinated; some are unmyelinated. Pain and temperature as well as the

Table 25.1 NERVE FIBER TYPE ORGANIZED BY RELATIVE DIAMETER

Relative diameter	Nerve fiber type	Function	Myelination	Conduction velocity (m/s)
Large	Aα	Somatic motor, touch and pressure	Yes	70–120
	1a	Muscle spindle afferents (proprioception–muscle length)	Yes	70–120
	1b	Golgi tendon organ afferents (proprioception–muscle tension)	Yes	70–120
Medium	Aβ	Touch and pressure	Yes	30–70
	Aγ	Spindle afferents (proprioception–muscle speed)	Yes	10–50
	II	Secondary afferents	Yes	30–70
Small	Aδ	Pain (fast, sharp) and temperature	Yes	4–30
	B	Preganglionic autonomic and visceral	Yes (light)	3–30

Table 25.1 CONTINUED

Relative diameter	Nerve fiber type	Function	Myelination	Conduction velocity (m/s)
	III	Pressure and pain	Yes	4–30
	C	Slow pain, postganglionic autonomic	No	0.5–2
	IV	Pain (slow, dull) and temperature	No	0.5–2

Adapted from Benarroch, Cutsforth-Gregory, and Flemming, *Mayo Clinic Medical Neurosciences: Organized by Neurologic System and Level.* Reprinted with permission from Oxford University Press © 2017.

autonomic nervous system are composed of small-diameter fibers, and postganglionic autonomic fibers tend to be unmyelinated. Although he also develops dysfunction of motor neurons as well as proprioception, which are both mediated by large-diameter fibers, this only occurs later in the disease course.

The onset of his symptoms, with early and severe pain and autonomic dysfunction, points to a neuropathy that involves the small-fiber peripheral nerves in the peripheral and autonomic nervous systems early on in the course of a chronic syndrome. This can be a clue to the underlying pathophysiology as to why these small fibers might be particularly vulnerable to his underlying disorder.

WHAT IS THE SYNDROMIC DIAGNOSIS?

He has chronic onset of peripheral and autonomic nervous system dysfunction with early/prominent small-fiber compared to large-fiber involvement.

WHAT IS THE ETIOLOGIC DIAGNOSIS?

We know this is a chronic disorder, so our etiologic differential diagnosis includes neurodegenerative diseases, genetic disorders, and drugs/toxins/metabolic. Given his young age and the fact that this doesn't fit any typical neurodegenerative disorder, we are left with this being either a genetic disorder or one caused by some sort of environmental exposure (such as a toxin or vitamin deficiency). In this case, a large laboratory work-up is surely indicated; however, we can use the principles we worked through earlier to vastly narrow down our differential diagnosis and the testing we order.

He presented with a chronically progressive neuropathy with key characteristics of both large- and small-fiber nerve involvement. There were early prominent features of small-fiber damage, as manifested by his autonomic dysfunction and length-dependent, severely painful neuropathy. We will need to target any work-up of these possible causes only to genetic or environmental diseases that cause this exact type of chronic polyneuropathy with notable early onset of small-fiber and autonomic involvement (syndromic diagnosis).

CONCLUSION

Ultimately, the pathologic diagnosis was transthyretin familial amyloid polyneuropathy (TTR-FAP), which was only diagnosed based on the results of genetic testing. This is a disease caused by a mutation in transthyretin (TTR), a serum protein that transports thyroxine and retinol. Pathogenic mutations cause mutant proteins to misfold and aggregate, forming insoluble fibrils that are deposited into various tissues. Patients can have variable presentations, such as deposition of insoluble fibrils in the heart causing cardiomyopathy. However, when the peripheral nerves are involved, it is common for small-fiber and autonomic involvement to occur early in the disease course.

Chapter 26

A man with difficulty climbing the stairs

A 55-year-old man developed pain in his lower extremities. He described approximately 1 year of constant, sharp pain that radiated from his waist down to his feet bilaterally. This pain was exacerbated with walking or standing up, and it was relieved with rest. He worked in construction, and he was having difficulty due to pain limiting his ability to walk or climb stairs. He also described low back pain and numbness/paresthesias around his groin, perineal area, buttocks, and feet for the past year. In addition, he had erectile dysfunction. He denied any bowel or bladder dysfunction. He wasn't able to elaborate further on the exact onset of symptoms, but they had not progressively worsened to his knowledge.

What had changed more recently, and the reason he sought medical evaluation, was that for the past 6 months he had developed new weakness. This initially began in his right arm. He noted difficulty raising his right arm above his head. However, his weakness progressed to involve all extremities to an equal degree. Although he already had difficulty walking and climbing stairs due to pain, he now believed that weakness was a contributing factor to his difficulty getting around. In addition, he endorsed diffuse, but mild, muscle cramping. Approximately 3 months after onset of his weakness, his primary care doctor recommended stopping his statin, which had been prescribed several years prior to onset of these symptoms. However, his symptoms (weakness and cramping) progressed despite cessation of statin therapy. He denied any recent illnesses or systemic symptoms. He denied any infectious or toxic exposures. There was no family history of neurologic disorders.

Before proceeding to his examination, take a minute to catalog his various symptoms. Is there one localization that puts everything together? Since he has chronic pain, could that be impacting his ability to estimate his degree of weakness? What patterns of weakness might you be looking for on your examination to help you localize the lesion?

On examination, mental status and cranial nerves were normal. Neck flexion and extension were both 4/5. Muscle bulk was decreased proximally in the bilateral upper extremities. Tone was normal. There were no spontaneous fasciculations or myokymia. He had scapular winging bilaterally. Shoulder abduction (after the first 15 degrees) was 2/5 bilaterally, biceps and triceps 4/5 bilaterally, and finger extensors 4/5 bilaterally. The rest of the intrinsic hand muscles had normal strength. Hip flexors and extensors were 4/5 bilaterally. Strength was otherwise full in the lower extremities. His reflexes were 1+ and symmetric throughout. His toes were down-going bilaterally. He had a positive straight-leg test bilaterally. He endorsed decreased sensation to light touch over his legs bilaterally in a nonspecific distribution. He had difficulty going from sitting to standing, but his stance and gait were normal.

WHAT IS THE PACE?

This one is tricky. Just like in our case of the woman with a vision loss (Chapter 5), there isn't a clear onset of his symptoms. He seems to have had the majority of his symptoms for at least a year, and many of his symptoms appear to be static. However, he also has newer weakness for the past 6 months that has progressively worsened. Is this a chronic process? Is this a subacute process? I would actually make the argument that it is difficult to definitively assign a *pace* without first understanding the localization. Let's move on to the localization and then return later to the pace.

WHAT IS THE LOCALIZATION?

His initial presenting symptoms were bilateral pain radiating down his legs, low back pain, saddle anesthesia, and erectile dysfunction. On examination, he had a positive straight-leg test bilaterally. All of these symptoms are highly suggestive of a lumbosacral radiculopathy. He has radiating radicular pain, a positive straight-leg test, and exacerbation of his symptoms with exertion (termed spinal claudication). These are all consistent with a lumbar radiculopathy. The addition of saddle anesthesia and erectile dysfunction indicates sacral dysfunction. Since we know he has dysfunction of the lumbar nerve roots, the etiology of his sacral dysfunction is likely the sacral nerve roots. Thus, by history and exam, he has a lumbosacral radiculopathy. There is little doubt about that localization. Can a lumbosacral radiculopathy explain his pattern of weakness?

Now things get a bit tricky. We suspect he has a lumbosacral radiculopathy, but we also know he has weakness in the upper and lower extremities. The weakness in his upper extremities is clearly not due to a lumbosacral radiculopathy. However, could it be due to a cervical radiculopathy? Perhaps he has both a lumbosacral radiculopathy *and* a cervical radiculopathy due to severe degenerative disease of the spine. That would be parsimonious and follow Occam's razor. Does his pattern or topography of weakness fit with that of a radiculopathy?

Let's start with the lower extremities. Multiple radiculopathies could cause us to have a difficult time discerning a specific pattern of weakness on examination. However, we would still expect to see involvement of both proximal and distal muscle groups in most lumbar radiculopathies. For example, hip extensor weakness, if due to a radiculopathy, would be associated with L4 or L5 nerve root dysfunction. In this case, we would expect varying degrees of weakness in the distal lower extremities (dorsiflexion, great toe extension, etc.). Since this is absent, the localization of his weakness in his lower extremities to a lumbar radiculopathy is less likely. Likewise, he has profound weakness proximally in the arms as well as the neck, but he has relative preservation of strength of the distal upper extremities. This topography of his weakness is identical in all extremities. He has much more severe proximal versus distal muscle weakness, which is more consistent with a myopathy than a radiculopathy.

The topography of weakness is critical to localization of peripheral nervous system disorders. Whether it is a proximal (or limb-girdle pattern) as described earlier, bulbar/facial weakness, ocular weakness, or other pattern, the topography gives us a tremendous amount of information regarding the underlying pathophysiology. Why there are differences in the topographic patterns of muscle weakness in different myopathies is unknown. There are various hypotheses, such as variations in muscle fiber type, size, and metabolic factors. However, what is clear in this case is that the pattern of weakness he presents with is most definitively myopathic.

Thus, our localization is *both* a lumbosacral radiculopathy *and* a myopathy. Let's go back to the pace.

WHAT IS THE PACE?

Or should we say paces? He presented with 1 year of static symptoms attributed to a lumbosacral radiculopathy. This is most consistent with a chronic pace. However, he also presented with progressive weakness over months attributed to a myopathy. This is most consistent with a subacute course of illness.

WHAT IS THE SYNDROMIC DIAGNOSIS?

How can we reconcile his presentation with a single lesion? The answer is that we can't. Occam's razor fails us in this case. Hickam's dictum, "a [patient] can have as many diseases as he [or she] damn well pleases," prevails over the diagnostic parsimony of Occam's razor. In this case, using the techniques of *pace* and *localization* makes that obvious. Let's tackle each syndrome independently.

He presents with syndromic diagnoses of a chronic lumbosacral radiculopathy and a subacute myopathy.

WHAT IS THE ETIOLOGIC DIAGNOSIS?

Potential etiologic diagnoses of his lumbosacral radiculopathy include genetic, neurodegenerative, neoplastic, structural, and toxic/metabolic causes. Theoretically, we could go through the exercise of trying to identify various pathologic diagnoses within

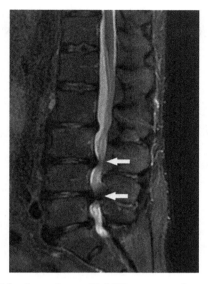

Figure 26.1. MRI lumbar spine sagittal T2 sequence shows severe canal and foraminal stenosis at multiple levels (*arrows*).

these categories. Practically, the initial work-up for a patient presenting with low back pain and radicular symptoms would be to obtain imaging, which is what was done and shown here in Figure 26.1.

MRI of his lumbar spine showed severe canal and foraminal stenosis at multiple levels, resulting in near-complete thecal sac effacement and impingement on the bilateral L4 and L5 nerve roots causing swelling in the roots. Due to these findings, he was taken for surgical decompression with improvement in many of the symptoms attributed to his lumbosacral radiculopathy.

Now, let's tackle his subacute onset of proximal muscle weakness most likely due to a myopathy. Additional work-up revealed a markedly elevated CK of 10,000. In addition, an MRI revealed diffuse, symmetric muscular edema consistent with myositis (Figure 26.2).

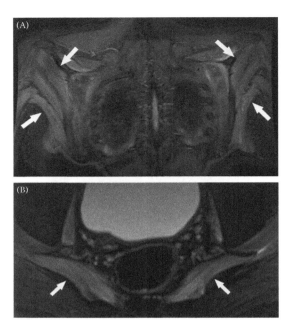

Figure 26.2. (**A**) MRI of the bilateral upper extremities STIR sequence shows diffuse abnormal edema (*arrows*) of multiple muscle groups. (**B**) MRI of the bilateral lower extremities T2 sequence shows similar features of edema in multiple muscle groups (*arrows*). Enhancement of multiple muscle groups not shown.

The potential etiologic diagnoses for a subacute course of disease include infectious, inflammatory, neoplastic, and toxic/metabolic disorders. Indeed, there are numerous causes of acquired myopathies. Based on his lack of systemic illness and reported exposures, we might consider infectious and toxic/metabolic disorders less likely. These are not ruled out, but the context makes an immune-mediated myopathy (inflammatory myositis) the most likely etiologic diagnosis.

CONCLUSION

Ultimately, his diagnosis was made after a muscle biopsy and a blood test. A muscle biopsy of his left deltoid revealed necrotic and regenerating fibers without inflammatory cell infiltrate consistent with an acute necrotizing myopathy. This was consistent with an immune-mediated myopathic process.

Statins can cause direct myopathic toxicity (ranging from mildly elevated CK to, rarely, rhabdomyolysis). However, in rare cases, and through an independent mechanism, they can trigger the formation of anti-HMG-CoA reductase autoantibodies, which our patient tested positive for with a highly elevated titer. This results in an immune-mediated necrotizing myopathy, which was the final pathologic diagnosis of his myopathy. This myopathy typically persists despite cessation of statin use and requires immune treatment.

Chapter 27

A man with pain in his arms

A 60-year-old right-handed man presented with pain in his right arm. His symptoms initially began with abrupt onset of burning pain radiating from the neck down the lateral aspect of his right arm. This was associated with numbness as well as some weakness with right elbow flexion. He denied any trauma or abnormal activities. Over the next few weeks, the pain and weakness worsened, and he developed difficulty writing, typing, and opening jars. He also had difficulty reaching for items high on a shelf or lifting his arm up to shampoo his hair. He had an MRI (Figure 27.1) that showed severe neuroforaminal stenosis at C4–C5 and C5–C6. Due to these findings and his symptoms, he underwent decompressive surgery. The radiating pain down his right arm improved after the surgery, but his weakness remained. He had mild pain over both of his shoulders and his neck. In addition, he developed numbness and painful paresthesias in his left hand. Finally, he developed weakness in the left hand as well, which led to him having to use specialized tools to help with everyday activities, such as flossing. He denied any lower extremity symptoms or bowel/bladder dysfunction.

What is your initial hypothesis as to whether the lesions are central or peripheral, and why? Based on that hypothesis, what components of the exam will we need to expand compared to the typical neurologic screening exam?

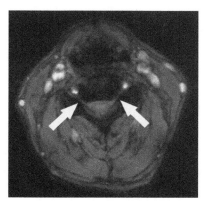

Figure 27.1. MRI cervical spine axial GRE sequence obtained preoperatively shows severe neuroforaminal stenosis (*arrows*) at C4–C5 and C5–C6 bilaterally (one representative cross-section shown).

His neurologic examination was notable for normal mental status and cranial nerves. He had decreased muscle bulk in his distal right upper extremity. There were also a few scattered fasciculations, and his muscle tone was normal or decreased throughout. He had bilateral scapular winging, worse on the right compared to the left. Strength testing in the right upper extremity revealed weakness with right shoulder abduction, flexion, internal rotation, and external rotation. He had bilateral weakness with elbow flexion and supination. He had a complete wrist drop on the right, and he was only anti-gravity with wrist extension on the left. Wrist flexion was weak bilaterally. The intrinsic muscles of the hands were also weak bilaterally, generally the right side more so than the left. His sensory examination showed diminished sensation to pinprick, light touch, and temperature scattered throughout his bilateral upper extremities. His reflexes were absent bilaterally at the triceps, biceps, and brachioradialis. Strength, sensation, and reflexes were all normal in the bilateral lower extremities. His gait was normal.

WHAT IS THE PACE?

All we have to work with for this case is that the onset of his pain was "abrupt." That likely means that the onset was either hyperacute or acute, but we can't say for sure. However, his symptoms progressed over the subsequent weeks to months, which is consistent with a subacute pace of symptoms. There seems to be both a hyperacute/acute presentation and a subacute worsening.

WHAT IS THE LOCALIZATION?

First, let's identify if the lesion(s) is in the central or peripheral nervous system. He presents with weakness, sensory loss, and diminished reflexes in a stepwise fashion that is completely isolated to his bilateral upper extremities. There is a notable lack of lower extremity involvement. He has some scattered fasciculations, decreased tone, and diminished reflexes. All of these point to a problem that localizes to the peripheral nervous system, but where?

We can easily rule out a muscle or neuromuscular junction disorder, since he has both motor and sensory dysfunction. Thus, we are left with a problem that lies somewhere between the spinal roots (radiculopathy or polyradiculopathy) and peripheral nerves (polyneuropathy or mononeuropathy) and everything in between (dorsal root ganglionopathy or plexopathy). The *topography* of his symptoms can help us narrow down his localization and clinical syndrome. Is there a pattern to his neurologic deficits (motor, sensory, reflexes) that fits a classic neuropathy or radiculopathy?

A polyneuropathy tends to be a more generalized process that is typically symmetrical and length-dependent. Because of this, symptom onset is typically in the distal lower extremities. That pattern does not fit this case.

A mononeuropathy manifests as weakness and/or sensory loss isolated to the distribution of a single nerve. This must be distinguished from a radiculopathy, which can present with substantial clinical overlap, but it can't be the case here. There is widespread dysfunction in both arms in the territory of many nerves.

For the same reason, a single radiculopathy is not possible. However, a polyradiculopathy or multiple mononeuropathies (mononeuritis multiplex) could be the possible localization. When we examine a patient several months into an illness, many of these disorders can start to appear quite similar if they have widespread involvement. However, even in this case, the pattern was always confusing and did not conform to any specific territory even at the onset.

It is precisely that non-localizable pattern of his symptoms that makes a plexopathy the most likely diagnosis. Plexopathies typically cause widespread motor and sensory involvement that doesn't fit the pattern of any one nerve or root. For example, our patient had scapular winging, caused by weakness of the serratus anterior, which is innervated by the long thoracic nerve (C5–C7). He also had weakness of the intrinsic hand muscles, indicating weakness of C8–T1. His proximal and distal weakness and sensory loss involving multiple nerves and roots without an apparent radicular or neuropathic pattern are most consistent with a plexopathy.

WHAT IS THE SYNDROMIC DIAGNOSIS?

He presented with hyperacute/acute onset of pain followed by subacute development of weakness and sensory loss in a stepwise fashion in the bilateral upper extremities consistent with bilateral brachial plexopathies. That is a mouthful!

WHAT IS THE ETIOLOGIC DIAGNOSIS?

If we follow our initial guidelines, then we can't rule out much, since the pace of disease seems to be a possible combination of hyperacute/acute and subacute.

Frequently, lesions of the brachial plexus are due to some form of mechanical trauma, whether it be due to a fall, motor vehicle collision, or prolonged traction during a surgery. However, there is no *context* of an extrinsic trauma. Brachial plexus injuries can also be due to internal trauma or compression, such as Pancoast syndrome or thoracic outlet syndrome. Presumably, that would be seen on imaging (normal, and not included). There is also an association of plexopathies and malignancy, which can be secondary to mass effect and tumor infiltration or radiation. Again, the context or imaging findings are not present. What else can cause bilateral or recurrent plexopathies? Is our localization or syndrome incorrect?

ADDITIONAL INFORMATION

Numerous laboratory studies were sent off to evaluate for acquired (infectious, inflammatory, toxic/metabolic) causes of polyradiculopathies or neuropathies. All of these studies were normal. If our localization was wrong and he did not have a plexopathy and his symptoms were instead due to a polyradiculopathy or polyneuropathy, we still did not find an etiology with our work-up.

CONCLUSION

Quite definitively, he did not have a chronic onset of symptoms, although this was ultimately due to a genetic condition. His case breaks the guidelines I established at the beginning of the book. Although the pace did not follow the rules and could have led us astray, the localization was specific enough for us to arrive at the diagnosis. If you search for recurrent or bilateral brachial plexopathy online, you will find his diagnosis among your search results.

He was diagnosed with hereditary neuralgic amyotrophy (HNA), which is an autosomal dominant disorder that presents with recurrent plexopathies (typically brachial, not lumbosacral). Some patients can have cranial nerve or autonomic symptoms or dysmorphic facial features. HNA is caused by mutations in septins, which are hetero-oligomeric GTP-binding proteins essential for microtubule-dependent cell processes.

Interestingly, after the patient was told of the possibility that he had a genetic disorder, he spoke to his family to see if anybody else had experienced similar symptoms. He had not provided this information initially, but his father suffered from recurrent dropped feet, his sister wore a brace because of a wrist drop, and his brother had recurrent episodes of wrist drop over several decades. The differential diagnosis and localization we generated ultimately led to a diagnosis in his other family members.

This is likely a diagnosis that is impossible to make without the appropriate localization, but once we identify the localization, we can make the correct diagnosis. That is the power of localization even when the pace is misleading.

Chapter 28

A man with painful, blurry vision

A 69-year-old man presented with eye swelling and pain. He was unsure of precisely when his symptoms started, but he said he had noticed that for at least "several" days prior to presentation his left eye appeared to be red, swollen, and painful. His vision from the left eye was blurry, but he wasn't sure if that was due to the excessive tearing he had from that side or was true vision loss. On the day of presentation, he developed vesicular lesions around the left eyelid and forehead. Within hours of developing the rash, he noted double vision with both eyes open in all directions of gaze. His double vision resolved when he closed one eye or the other. By the next day, the double vision was so severe that he kept his left eye completely shut so that he would be able to see.

As neurologists we frequently encounter patients who present with visual disturbance. Typically, but not always, these patients have seen an optometrist or ophthalmologist prior to our evaluation. In some ways, this makes our job easier. The optometrist/ophthalmologist has presumably already evaluated the patient for primary ocular disorders such as glaucoma or cataracts. Thus, we tend to encounter a patient population with visual disturbances that is enriched for neuro-ophthalmologic disorders, since most patients with primary ocular pathology have already been screened out. We must consider those primary ocular pathologies in our differential, but once those have been excluded, we are left with various neuro-ophthalmologic diseases. The first step at that point is typically determining whether there is dysfunction of the afferent (optic nerve) or efferent (extraocular muscles) pathways related to vision. That will help us to localize the lesion. What clues in the history might localize to afferent or efferent (or both) visual dysfunction?

On examination, he had a vesicular rash over the left eyelid and forehead. There was left upper eyelid ptosis with edema and mild hyperemia. In addition, he had 1 to 2 mm of proptosis on the left. He had diffuse conjunctival injection on the left with excessive lacrimation. Visual acuity was 20/50 OD (right eye) and 20/200 OS (left eye). He had anisocoria: His left pupil was larger than the right and poorly reactive to light. His pupil did not constrict with convergence. In addition, he had a left relative afferent pupillary defect. His extraocular movements were normal on the right. On the left, he had severe limitation of movement with supraduction, adduction, and infraduction. There was mild restriction of abduction of the left eye. He had painful dysesthesias over the forehead on the left side. The rest of his neurologic exam, including the remainder of his cranial nerves, was normal.

WHAT IS THE PACE?

Prior to the definitive onset of his neurologic symptoms (double vision), he had a prodrome of pain and rash. In this case, we could consider that to be the beginning of his symptoms, or we could "start the clock" with onset of his double vision. This is a mostly arbitrary decision. However, the description that within hours of onset of his rash he noted new double vision that wasn't there before is fairly definitive. His symptoms evolving over the course of hours (and maybe days) is consistent with an acute pace of disease.

WHAT IS THE LOCALIZATION?

Hopefully, there is no ambiguity that his signs and symptoms are consistent with dysfunction of the cranial nerves. For this case, our localization is restricted to identifying where the lesion is along the afferent and/or efferent pathways related to vision. This could be anywhere between the eye and orbit going back to the brainstem. Although that is a relatively small geographic space in the nervous system, there are many complex different potential pathologies that remain on the differential prior to identifying the specific anatomic syndrome. For example, an internuclear ophthalmoplegia is due to a lesion in the medial longitudinal fasciculus, but an isolated unilateral adduction deficit could be due to an infiltrative orbital process or partial third-nerve palsy. These conditions look strikingly similar on examination, but the differential diagnoses of these disorders are dramatically different. Thus, it is critical to perform a precise exam to help us appropriately localize the lesion.

This case can replicate the thought process of how to think like a neurologist to only a limited degree. Carefully examining this patient takes practice, and there is no substitute for learning the subtleties of how to identify various ophthalmopareses. Read the exam again, and try to visualize how you would test the various actions. Now, let's go stepwise through the exam to determine which actions are affected and, in turn, which cranial nerves might be involved. I say "might" since an intraorbital process directly affecting the muscles themselves (rather than the nerves) could also cause similar restrictions in eye movement.

First, he had decreased visual acuity OS, and he had anisocoria. His left pupil was dilated and minimally reactive to light. This could be due to damage to the parasympathetic fibers that travel with the third cranial nerve and innervate the sphincter pupillae and ciliary muscles (efferent). In fact, it does look like that is the case (as his pupil does not constrict with convergence). However, he also has a relative afferent pupillary defect. This indicates damage to the afferent visual input (optic nerve).

As we mentioned, there is damage to the parasympathetic fibers of the oculomotor (III) nerve. What are its other actions, and are they intact? The oculomotor nerve also innervates the muscles responsible for supraduction, infraduction, and adduction, which are all impaired. In addition, he has ptosis. Taken all together, this indicates an oculomotor nerve palsy. Although these various deficits could localize to a muscle or neuromuscular process (such as myasthenia), the pupillary involvement helps us localize his deficits to a third-nerve palsy.

Is there evidence of a trochlear (IV) nerve palsy? This is hard to definitively say in this example due to the severe third-nerve palsy. The trochlear nerve innervates the superior oblique, which intorts, depresses, and abducts the eye.

Is there an abducens (VI) nerve palsy? There is slightly restricted abduction, which indicates a paresis of the lateral rectus muscle. This could be due to an abducens nerve palsy.

Lastly, he also has sensory changes over the forehead. The sensory innervation for this area is the V1 division of the trigeminal nerve.

Now that we have gone through all of his findings, let's list them out together. He has deficits involving cranial nerves II, III, (IV?), V1, and VI. Is there one location that can cause dysfunction in all of these cranial nerves simultaneously?

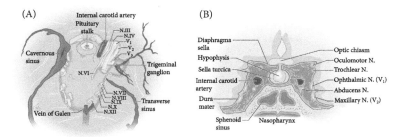

Figure 28.1. Drawing of a coronal cross-section of the cavernous sinus showing the structures traversing through and around the cavernous sinus. (A) Depiction of cranial nerve roots emerging from the brainstem in relationship to other major structures and (B) cross-section of cranial nerves and other major structures in and adjacent to the cavernous sinus. *Republished with permission of McGraw Hill LLC, from Adams and Victor's Principles of Neurology, Ropper, Allan H., Martin A. Samuels, Joshua P. Klein, and Sashank Prasad, 11th edition, 2019; permission conveyed through Copyright Clearance Center, Inc.*

Intracranially, these nerves are in relatively disparate locations. A single intracranial lesion would need to be quite large or involve large parts of the brainstem to cause these findings. Without evidence of other signs or symptoms, it would be highly unlikely that we would find a large brainstem lesion. However, all of these nerves must converge on the orbit. They pass through various foramina (such as the superior orbital fissure and optic canal). This creates a choke point. At this point, you may want to reference Figure 28.1 and Table 28.1 to determine if this specific combination of cranial neuropathies can occur due to a single lesion.

WHAT IS THE SYNDROMIC DIAGNOSIS?

He presents with acute onset of dysfunction of cranial nerves II, III, (IV?), V1, and VI. These cranial nerves all simultaneously

Table 28.1 STRUCTURES INVOLVED IN ORBITAL APEX, SUPERIOR
ORBITAL FISSURE, AND CAVERNOUS SINUS SYNDROMES

Structure	Orbital apex	Superior orbital fissure	Cavernous sinus
Cranial nerve II	+	−	−[a]
Cranial nerve III	+	+	+
Cranial nerve IV	+	+	+
Cranial nerve V1	+	+	+
Cranial nerve V2	−	−	+
Cranial nerve VI	+	+	+
Carotid artery	−	−	+

Abbreviations: +, involved; −, not involved.
[a] Can be indirectly involved
Adapted from Thurtell and Tomsak, *Neuro-Ophthalmology Second Edition*. Reprinted with permission from Oxford University Press © 2012.

pass through the apex of the orbit, and the constellation of symptoms caused by their dysfunction is known as orbital apex syndrome.

WHAT IS THE ETIOLOGIC DIAGNOSIS?

He presents with acute onset of orbital apex syndrome. Therefore, we expect our etiologic diagnosis to be due to either an infectious or inflammatory disorder in the orbital apex.

CONCLUSION

An MRI showed evidence of inflammation in the orbit (Figure 28.2).

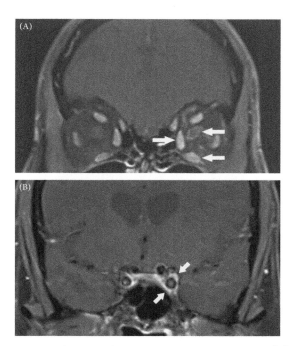

Figure 28.2. MRI orbit coronal T1 post-contrast images reveal (**A**) mild enlargement of the medial and inferior rectus muscles (*arrows*), enhancement around the optic nerve sheath on the left, and (**B**) enhancement extends back to the orbital apex and superior left cavernous sinus (*arrows*).

The context in this case helps us make the diagnosis. He had a vesicular rash in the distribution of V1. This is consistent with zoster ophthalmicus, which is caused by reactivation of varicella-zoster virus from sensory ganglia. It travels along neurons and erupts as a vesicular skin rash in the distribution of the nerve it infects. Rarely, herpes zoster ophthalmicus can be complicated by dysfunction of other cranial nerves, as in this case, where it caused orbital apex syndrome. The exact pathophysiology is unclear, but it could be due to direct viral cytopathic effect. He was treated with antivirals and systemic as well as topical steroids. His neurologic exam improved significantly after starting treatment.

Chapter 29

A woman with blurry vision and difficulty driving

A 39-year-old right-handed woman was admitted to the hospital after developing visual symptoms while driving. She described the sudden onset of blurry or hazy vision in her left eye, which was associated with left-sided numbness (face, arm, and leg) and dysarthria. She was unable to hold the steering wheel with her left hand or manipulate the gas pedal if she tried to use her left foot. These symptoms resolved within a few hours. Work-up at that time, including MRI brain (discussed later), was unrevealing for a cause of her presentation.

She was subsequently admitted to the hospital again at the age of 46 after presenting with sudden onset of bilateral blurred vision, which was present with either eye closed. Approximately 30 minutes later she developed numbness in both of her hands, which advanced up her arms. Ten minutes after she developed symptoms in her arms, she began having bilateral lower extremity weakness (worse on the right compared to the left). Her symptoms progressed to the point at which she could no longer ambulate. By the time she arrived at the hospital her symptoms had already begun improving.

Her prior medical history was notable for the onset of migraine headaches at the age of 33. She characterized the headaches as coming on over minutes to hours. The headaches were throbbing and associated with nausea and light sensitivity (photophobia) and lasted up to 72 hours at a time. She would occasionally have a visual aura. Around the time of headache onset she also developed hypertension. A work-up of secondary causes of hypertension was unremarkable.

What are the characteristics of the two episodes of transient neurologic dysfunction? Which one seems to have a more straightforward syndrome and localization, and which one is more complex? When a patient has transient neurologic dysfunction, their symptoms can be fleeting. Because of this, they might have few signs on their neurologic exam to help localize the lesion. When that is the case, the history might be all we have to go by to help localize the lesion if the exam is unremarkable.

On examination at the time of her initial episode, she was found to have left-sided sensory loss to touch (face, arm, and leg) and mild left arm and leg weakness with a pronator drift. Her examination at the hospital after her second episode was documented as normal. An examination done several months after the second event was notable for normal mental status, cranial nerve, motor, sensory, and cerebellar examinations. However, she had brisk reflexes on the right compared to the left, including positive Hoffmann's and Babinski's reflexes.

WHAT IS THE PACE?

This one is tricky. The events that led to each hospital admission are clearly hyperacute to acute. Her symptoms come on suddenly and resolve within hours. There is no progression of symptoms over the course of days. However, there also appears to be an additional more chronic aspect to her symptoms. Seemingly out of the blue, she developed several episodes of transient neurologic symptoms and new-onset migraines over the course of the past decade. In this case, the recurrent nature of transient neurologic symptoms is best described as a chronic time course of hyperacute events.

WHAT IS THE LOCALIZATION?

The localization of her symptoms has to be central and involving the brain given her history of headaches, dysarthria, and vision changes. Let's discuss her first presentation in more detail. She had symptoms involving left-sided numbness with dysarthria and inco-ordination/weakness. We thus need to put her lesion in an area of the CNS where the motor and sensory fibers to the face and body are traveling in close proximity.

Can the lesion be cortical? It is possible to have these deficits from a cortical lesion. However, to do so would require a very large hemispheric lesion. Remember, the cortical homunculus covers the midline of the parietal cortex from the level of the corpus callosum and wraps all the way along the outer parietal lobe down to the insular cortex. To have a lesion that large, we would expect other cortical deficits from a nondominant parietal lobe lesion to also be present, such as hemi-neglect (anosognosia), certain types of apraxia (learned, complex movements), or spatial disorientation.

Can the lesion be subcortical or in the deep gray structures (i.e., basal ganglia or thalamus)? The corticospinal tract descends from the cortex via the internal capsule on its way to the brainstem and spinal cord. Likewise, the sensory tracts ascend through the spinal cord, synapse in the thalamus, and then ascend through the internal capsule en route to the cortex. These axons carrying motor and sensory information to all parts of the body are compressed in close proximity. Here, information to the face, arm, and legs is in close proximity, so a single lesion can lead to a variety of more widespread symptoms. This is the localization of the so-called lacunar syndromes in stroke and fits quite nicely for our patient.

Can the lesion be found in the brainstem? In the brainstem, just as in the internal capsule and thalamus, information to various parts of the body is compressed into a small space, so large dramatic presentations are possible with only a small lesion. However, we don't see any "crossed findings" that we might expect to see in a brainstem lesion, where cranial nerve nuclei are ipsilateral to their output and fibers going to the body are contralateral to their output. In addition, we don't see any typical cranial nerve syndromes that would point to one particular part of the brainstem.

Based on her exam, we should expect her lesion to be located deep to the cortex within the arcuate fibers, internal capsule, or even thalamus.

CLINICAL COURSE AND ADDITIONAL INFORMATION

Since she presents to the emergency room with sudden onset of neurologic symptoms, we will look at her imaging studies earlier in this case than we have done in other cases in this book.

Her MRIs (Figure 29.1) did not show any evidence of acute stroke while she was symptomatic. However, the MRIs did show progressive accumulation of hyperintense lesions involving her deep white matter from her initial MRI to the next one obtained 7 years later. In addition, there was a single contrast-enhancing lesion

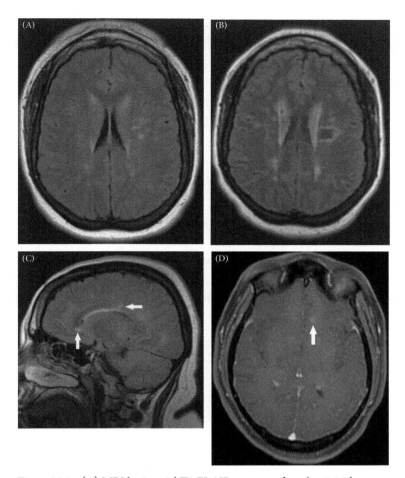

Figure 29.1. (**A**) MRI brain axial T2 FLAIR sequence from her initial presentation. (**B**) MRI brain axial T2 FLAIR sequence from her subsequent presentation shows increased number of hyperintense lesions in the deep white matter. (**C**) MRI brain sagittal T2 FLAIR from her subsequent presentation shows several perpendicularly oriented T2 hyperintense lesions (*arrows*) radiating off the corpus callosum. (**D**) MRI brain axial T1 post-contrast image from her subsequent presentation shows a left frontal enhancing lesion (*arrow*).

HOW TO THINK LIKE A NEUROLOGIST

present on her latest MRI. These findings were thought to potentially be consistent with demyelinating disease, such as multiple sclerosis, so she underwent an MRI of her cervical and thoracic spine, which were unremarkable. She also had a lumbar puncture to evaluate for various inflammatory and infectious conditions. CSF analysis was normal, including for the absence of oligoclonal bands.

WHAT IS THE SYNDROMIC DIAGNOSIS?

The ancillary data doesn't particularly help us, especially if you aren't already an expert in neuroradiology! Let's go back to our pace and localization to define the clinical syndrome. As we previously discussed, this is a chronic process that is punctuated by acute/hyperacute events that localizes to the deep cerebral hemispheres.

WHAT IS THE ETIOLOGIC DIAGNOSIS?

Let's put together the two paces to determine the potential etiologies of her presentation. The episodes of abrupt onset of neurologic dysfunction have a limited etiologic differential. These episodes of transient symptoms are *too fast* for an autoimmune or demyelinating disease. Her MRI clouds the picture. Even though her imaging might be consistent with an autoimmune demyelinating disease, her syndrome is not. Given the pace and localization of her deficits, the etiology of these episodes of hyperacute onset of symptoms must be vascular, even though we see no evidence of acute stroke on imaging to back up our theory.

She has recurrent episodes of transient neurologic dysfunction over a prolonged, chronic time period. Our list of chronic processes is relatively short: neurodegenerative diseases, congenital/genetic disorders, and drugs/toxins. Let's add the context. She isn't the typical demographic (too young) of what we might expect for neurodegenerative disease, and there isn't anything in her history to suggest drugs or toxin exposure. That means we are left with a suspicion for a congenital or genetic conditions. Putting all of this together, she has a chronic course of sudden, transient neurologic dysfunction due to ischemia. Using your search engine of choice, search for genetic disorders that cause increased risk of stroke and migraines, and you are likely to come up with the correct diagnosis as your top hit, or at least somewhere on the first page.

CONCLUSION

She was diagnosed with cerebral autosomal dominant arteriopathy with subcortical infarcts and leukoencephalopathy (CADASIL), which is an inherited condition that commonly causes ischemic strokes and migraines along with other symptoms such as cognitive decline, mood disturbances, and seizures. CADASIL is caused by a mutation in the NOTCH3 gene, which makes the Notch3 receptor protein found on the surface of vascular smooth muscle cells. Mutations in the Notch3 receptor protein cause damage to the vascular smooth muscles in the brain, which leads to the clinical phenotype.

Chapter 30

A woman with a tingling scalp

A 22-year-old woman presented with paresthesias approximately 1 week after developing a mild upper respiratory tract infection. The paresthesias involved her entire body, including her scalp and the inside of her mouth. In addition, she noted blurry vision, dizziness, and some mild gait instability. She presented to the emergency room the following day when her symptoms had not resolved. Over the course of that day, she lost the ability to walk, and her coordination became so impaired she couldn't feed herself with utensils. She ceased being able to speak due to weakness of her face and tongue. By 48 hours after symptom onset, she no longer had any verbal output. Her mother, who worked as a nurse, was adamant she was not speaking purely because of facial weakness and not aphasia. Due to the acute decline of her neurologic status, she was transferred to a tertiary referral center.

This history is dramatic. A young woman presents with a rapidly progressive neurologic syndrome after a recent upper respiratory infection. Over a relatively short period of time, she has severe neurologic deficits that have accrued at an alarming rate. Based on her history, what might you expect to find on her exam? What key features will you be looking for to confirm (or refute) your hypothesis?

The following examination occurred approximately 2.5 days into development of her neurologic symptoms. Her heart rate and blood pressure were fluctuating between severe hypotension and hypertension. She was awake, but she couldn't open her eyes due to severe ptosis. Although she couldn't speak, she could respond appropriately to multiple-choice questions with small nodding of her head. However, she could only answer simple questions, and her responses were abnormally delayed. Her pupils were 8 mm bilaterally and constricted to 5 mm with light. She had completely restricted up-gaze, partially limited right-gaze, limited down-gaze, and a right hypertropia. She had no facial movement whatsoever, and she couldn't stick her tongue out of her mouth or move it from side to side. She had minimal movement with attempted neck flexion and extension. Her tone was flaccid, except for her right upper extremity, which had increased tone. Strength in all extremities was at least better than anti-gravity, but it was difficult to assess exactly how much weakness she had, as she had severe sensory loss. She had complete absence of all sensory modalities—pinprick, temperature, vibration, and proprioception—over her entire body. Her movements were uncoordinated and ataxic.

Within an hour of the above examination, she became unresponsive and was intubated.

WHAT IS THE PACE?

She developed neurologic symptoms over hours to days, which is consistent with acute onset of disease.

WHAT IS THE LOCALIZATION?

There is a lot going on, both in her history and examination. For this case, given the multitude of signs and symptoms, let's try to break everything down by the major components or domains of the neurologic exam: mental status, cranial nerves, sensory and motor examination, reflexes, coordination, and gait.

Is there evidence of a change in mental status? Testing for mental status changes in a critically ill patient can be tricky, especially in one with bilateral ptosis or eyelid apraxia (not a true apraxia, but a condition frequently seen after nondominant parietal lobe injury), where the patient might appear to be asleep or unarousable but is actually awake. In her case, she could answer questions initially, but her responses were delayed and limited. She then became unresponsive. Her syndrome includes alteration of consciousness. As discussed in Chapter 7, this can be secondary to either brainstem, thalamic, or bilateral cortical involvement.

Is there evidence of cranial nerve dysfunction? Most definitely, yes. She has severe restriction of extraocular movements with almost no movement. She has bifacial diplegia. Her bulbar muscles are paralyzed. This could be secondary to either widespread brainstem involvement or dysfunction of the cranial nerves after they emerge from the brainstem.

Is there evidence of motor dysfunction? Yes, but oddly, it seems to be more preserved than other domains. She is at least better than antigravity strength. She does have involvement of neck flexion and extension. She has flaccid tone throughout, except for one extremity that has increased tone. That is a little bit peculiar. Decreased tone indicates the localization of her motor dysfunction is peripheral (as well as neck weakness), whereas the one extremity with increased tone indicates the localization could also be in the central nervous system.

Is there evidence of sensory dysfunction? If it weren't for her severe cranial neuropathies, this would be the most striking clinical feature. She has complete sensory loss throughout her entire body, and all sensory modalities are affected. Even by history, the inside of her mouth was involved on the first day of symptom onset. This argues in favor of dysfunction of the peripheral (and trigeminal) nerves.

Coordination was difficult to test, due to her severe sensory loss. When sensory loss is so severe, patients develop what is referred to as a *sensory ataxia* when they have profound proprioceptive loss. One way to distinguish proprioceptive versus cerebellar dysfunction as the cause of ataxia is to test the patient with eyes open and eyes closed. Sensory ataxia should improve with eyes open since visual input tells the brain where the limbs are in space (the Romberg test uses this principle or testing finger-to-nose with eyes open and eyes closed). Cerebellar ataxia should not be noticeably different with eyes open or eyes closed. However, in extreme cases like this, especially with her severe ptosis, it was difficult to determine if she also had cerebellar dysfunction. We were unable to assess gait due to her clinical instability.

ADDITIONAL INFORMATION

MRI brain and spine and CSF results were normal.

Some of you may have noticed that I did not mention or discuss her reflexes. That was intentional. What was the first thought after you read her history, or maybe even just the first line of her history? *A 22-year-old woman developed paresthesias and lost the ability to walk after an infection.* I imagine Guillain–Barré syndrome (GBS) jumped into many of your minds. For those of you reading along who are more advanced in your training, you might have even thought of some of the variants of GBS, such as Miller Fisher variant, which causes ophthalmoplegia and ataxia. If this were GBS (or one of its variants), do you expect her to have diminished/absent reflexes, normal reflexes, or hyperreflexia?

On exam, she had pathologic *hyperreflexia*. She had pectoral reflexes, crossed adductors, and sustained clonus at her ankles, and her toes were up-going bilaterally.

Now what? This can't be GBS, as you would expect areflexia, but what is it? Let's take stock of each affected domain and its possible localizations.

WHAT IS THE LOCALIZATION?

She presents with encephalopathy, cranial nerve dysfunction, motor dysfunction, sensory loss, and hyperreflexia. Can we come up with a single lesion to explain all of her deficits? Kind of, but not really. She has some features that indicate peripheral nervous system dysfunction, such as her motor exam and the profound degree of sensory loss indicating a polyneuropathy or polyradiculoneuropathy. Her cranial nerve deficits could be due to a brainstem lesion, but they could also be "peripheral" deficits if the dysfunction was due to injury to the nerves after they leave the brainstem. However, she also has signs and symptoms of central nervous system dysfunction. She has encephalopathy and decreased arousal as well as diffuse hyperreflexia. What's the only part of the nervous system where we can get altered arousal, cranial neuropathies, widespread motor/sensory dysfunction, and hyperreflexia? The brainstem.

WHAT IS THE SYNDROMIC DIAGNOSIS?

She presents with acute onset of brainstem and peripheral polyneuropathy or polyradiculoneuropathy.

WHAT IS THE ETIOLOGIC DIAGNOSIS?

Since the pace of symptoms is acute, our potential etiologic diagnoses include either infectious or inflammatory disorders. There is a very short list of disorders associated with rapidly progressive brainstem encephalitis, many of which are potentially fatal if untreated, such as *Listeria monocytogenes*. The list of diseases that cause a rapidly progressive brainstem encephalitis and polyneuropathy is even shorter.

CONCLUSION

Ultimately, she was diagnosed with Bickerstaff brainstem encephalitis. This disorder was first published in 1951 by Bickerstaff and Cloake, who described three patients with encephalopathy, ophthalmoplegia, and ataxia. They localized this syndrome as a mesencephalitis (inflammation of the midbrain) or rhomboencephalitis (inflammation of the pons, medulla, and cerebellum). Since that time, there has been some debate in the literature whether this is a distinct diagnosis from Miller Fisher variant GBS, or whether both disorders are the same disease with varying peripheral versus central nervous system involvement. The major difference in clinical syndromes between Miller Fisher variant

GBS and Bickerstaff brainstem encephalitis is encephalopathy. This patient's case argues for the theory that Miller Fisher variant GBS and Bickerstaff brainstem encephalitis are simply different phenotypes of the same disease, given her features of both central and peripheral nerve involvement.

Both Miller Fisher variant GBS and Bickerstaff brainstem encephalitis have an association with anti-GQ1b antibodies. Our patient had strikingly high titers, which confirmed the diagnosis. Remember, her MRI and lumbar puncture were both normal. This case could only be solved in the emergency setting using pace and localization. Thankfully, she made a full recovery after receiving treatment with plasma exchange and rituximab.

This case highlights the power of an unexpected exam finding. In the end, for those of you who immediately thought "GBS" when you read the initial history, you weren't too far off the ultimate diagnosis. However, a simple up-going toe or brisk reflex dramatically changes the localization and differential diagnosis.

INDEX

Tables and figures are indicated by *t* and *f* following the page number.

INDEX

myasthenia gravis, 144–145
myeloneuropathy, 152–153
myopathy, 195–196, 197–199
myositis, 197–198, 198f

NA (nucleus ambiguous), 180f
neck pain, in bacterial meningitis, 21, 23
necrotizing myopathy, immune-mediated,
     192–199
   etiologic diagnosis, 196–198, 197f, 198f
   localization, 194–196
   pace, 194, 196
   pathologic diagnosis, 199
   presentation of symptoms, 192–193
   syndromic diagnosis, 196
nerve fiber types, 187–189, 188t
nervous system, localizing lesions in. See
     localization
neuroborreliosis, 95–96
neuromyelitis optica spectrum disorder
     (NMOSD), 80–88
   etiologic diagnosis, 87
   localization, 82–86, 83f, 84f, 85f
   MRI results, 87, 88f
   pace, 81
   pathologic diagnosis, 88
   presentation of symptoms, 80–81
   syndromic diagnosis, 87
neuropathy, thoracic, 89–91, 94, 95–96
non-fluent aphasia, 21, 23
non-pruritic, erythematous rash, 89, 95–96
NOTCH3 gene, mutation in, 221
nucleus ambiguous (NA), 180f
nucleus of the tractus solitarius (NTS), 179,
     180f
nystagmus, direction-changing, 63, 64, 169,
     170

Occam's razor, 11
oculomotor nerve palsy, 210
oculovestibular incoordination, 65f
onset of symptoms. See pace
orbital apex syndrome, 207–214
   etiologic diagnosis, 212
   localization, 209–211, 211f
   MRI, 213f
   pace, 208–209

pathologic diagnosis, 213–214
presentation of symptoms, 207–208
structures involved in, 212t
syndromic diagnosis, 211–212
orthopnea, 141, 147
otitis media, 21

pace
   acute symptoms, 3–4, 7t
   categories, 3–6
   categories of disease, 6, 7t
   caveats, 4–5
   chronic symptoms, 4, 7t
   in clinical reasoning formula, 1
   defined, 2–3
   defining prior to localization, 11–12
   hyperacute symptoms, 3, 7t
   subacute symptoms, 4, 7t
   with unknown onset, 70f
pain
   in hereditary neuralgic amyotrophy,
      200–206
   in herpes zoster ophthalmicus, 207–214
   in immune-mediated necrotizing
      myopathy, 192–193, 194
   in transthyretin familial amyloid
      polyneuropathy, 184–191
palpebral oculogyric reflex, 92
papilledema, 114, 156
paraneoplastic cerebellar degeneration,
     62–67
   differential diagnosis, 66–67
   etiologic diagnosis, 66–67
   localization, 64–65
   pace, 64
   presentation of symptoms, 62–63
   syndromic diagnosis, 66
paraneoplastic syndrome, 130
parkinsonism, 78
pathologic diagnosis, defined, 13. See also
      specific diseases and syndromes
Percheron, artery of, 60–61
peripheral nervous system, lesions in, 30, 144
peripheral neuropathy, 144, 186–187
personality changes, 122
phrenic nerve dysfunction, 147
pinpoint pupils, 107–108, 109

236